What started out as simple reprint of Allen Cohen's "Childbirth Is Ecstasy" book turned into a four year project. Allen was very fond of this book and near the end of his life he would look at it often and that prompted my desire to help get this book back in print.

It started with an 8 month search for a copy of the book that we could take apart and scan for the reissue. Then in the process of going through Allen's documents we located a packet of photos and elements of the original book and that made us want to use the original photos to give the book the sharpest image and reprint possible. We originally thought we had most of the photos but when we scanned them we quickly realized that we only had half of them. At this point we thought we would have to use half of the photos and half book scans to complete it. Then during an Oracle get together Stephen Walzer mentioned that he still had the original negatives for the photos. So over the next year Stephen searched for the photos and one day I got a call that he had found them and he would put them in a safe place. So we thought at that point we would have all of the original photos but it turned out that the place was too safe and he could not remember where they were. It seems as fast as they were found they disappeared into the void again. Stephen passed away during the making of this reissue and all hope of finding those negatives was lost. Then one night during an online search on the book we realized the original elements for the book were in the archives at the San Francisco Library. Allen's widow Ann spent the next year and a half trying to get copies of the photos from the archives. Finally when we were about to give up they located them and scanned the original photos for us. It turned out Allen had half of the photos in his possession and the other half he had donated to the library with some other documents. After years of looking we had restored all of the original elements of the book.

We were now ready to work on the restoration of the book. At this point it was our desire to not use any scans and rebuild the book from the ground up. Ann Cohen retyped the entire text so the pages could be layed out again. John Taylor took on the pains-taking task of re-laying the type exactly as it was in the original book. Then the scans of the photos had to be completely restored. It turned out that the photos from the San Francisco library were in worse shape than the ones Allen had in his possession. John restored each photograph removing all of the dust and scratches that had happened in the 40 years since the first issue of this book. All of the photos and text have been re-layed to give you an exact replica of the original book. After 4 years the book has been completely restored and the version you are now holding surpasses the quality of the original book.

I hope you enjoy this 2011 edition Allen's Cohen and Stephen Walzer's Book Childbirth is Ecstasy. I know if Allen was here he would be proud to see it back in print

Enjoy,

Karl F Anderson II
Global Recording Artists January, 2011

I was honored that Karl asked me to help work on restoring this book. I had previously designed the multi-page program for the "40th Anniversary of the Summer of Love" event which took place in Golden Gate Park in San Francisco during the summer of 2007. At that time I had the fortune to meet Ann Cohen, Allen's widow, and to use some of her archives as part of the program. This has been a labor, but one of love and devotion especially to Ann. Her spirit and dedication to celebrating Allen's life and very public career as writer, poet, entrepreneur, and one of the progenitors of the late "Beat Movement" of the mid sixties, is without parallel.
It is with genuine pride that we present this seminal work by Allen Cohen and Steve Walzer as it was originally published some 40 years ago. I hope you enjoy it as much as I did as part of the project team.

John Taylor January 2011

O great Mother-Muse of the universe of generated forms

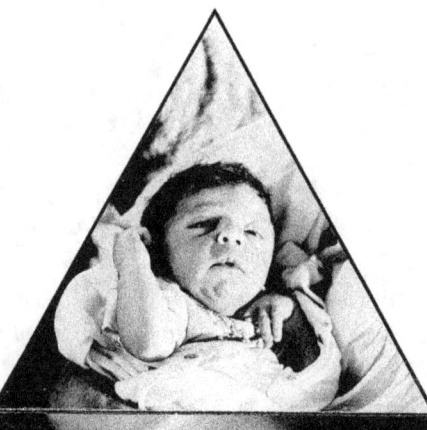

O courage beauty & love of human mothers

O perfection of the body-mandala through which we appear

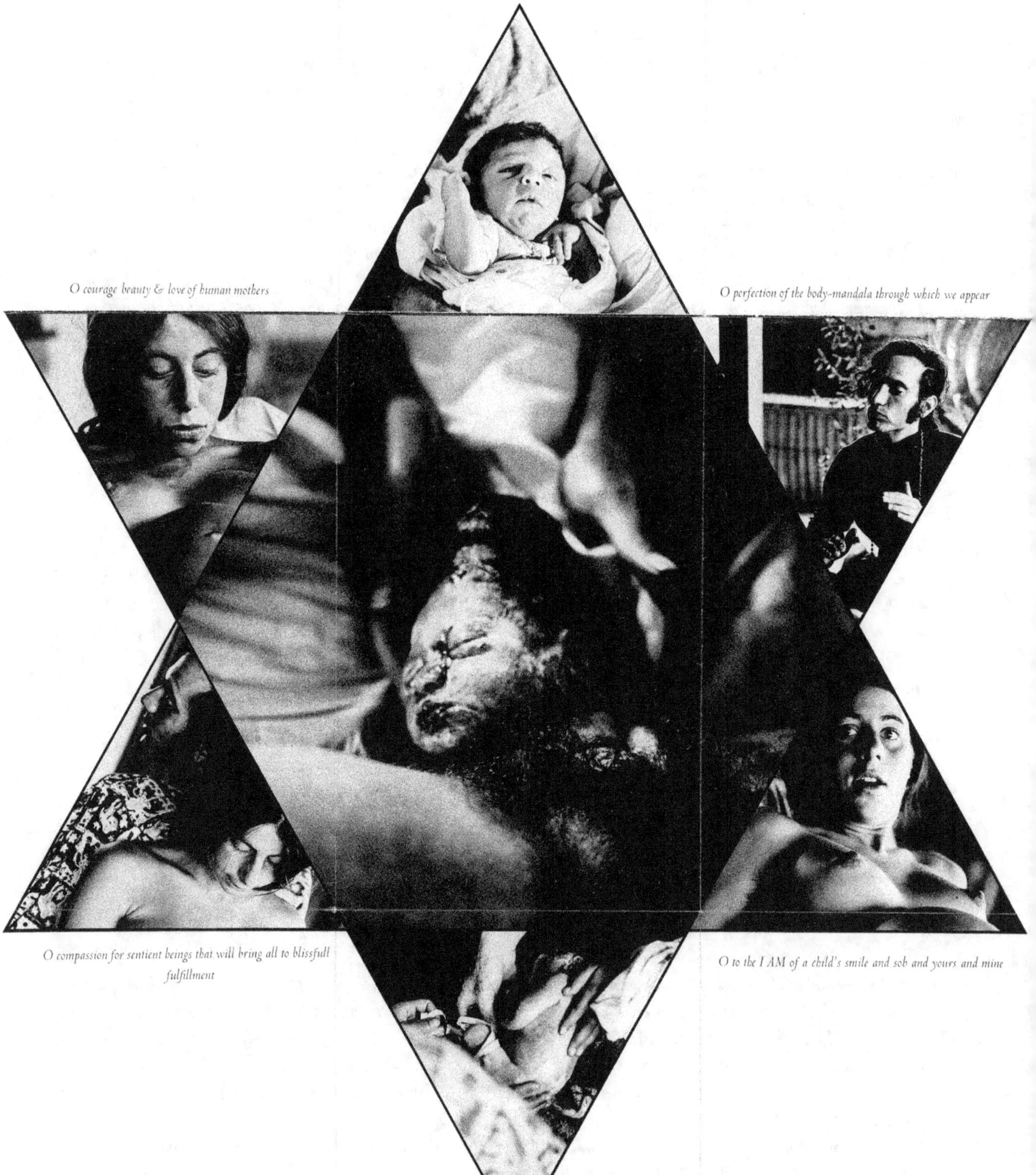

O compassion for sentient beings that will bring all to blissfull fulfillment

O to the I AM of a child's smile and sob and yours and mine

NOW & NOW & NOW

How do forty one years slip away so easily? Now, it seems like no trouble at all. Memory is a crazy thing! When I carried my children around in my belly, I promised myself that I would not forget the amazing feelings and sense of being kissed every moment, by God, in an extraordinary way.
I can draw on those memories when I need them because they are stored in the cells and tissues of my body. Just as the moment that River's head came out and then his shoulders, I can't help but recall the absolute ecstasy of the immergence of a new human being into my world. This experience was enormous in every way. It was physical, mental, spiritual, and emotional.

It is sad to me to think of all of the mothers starting out today who don't know the gifts that are there for them. Many women are lured into epidurals and many think that c-sections are the 'easy' way out. We live in a time where being unhappy requires medication, being anxious is not acceptable, children are given all sorts of drugs for attention deficit, and in general, our culture is becoming more and more alienated from natural experiences

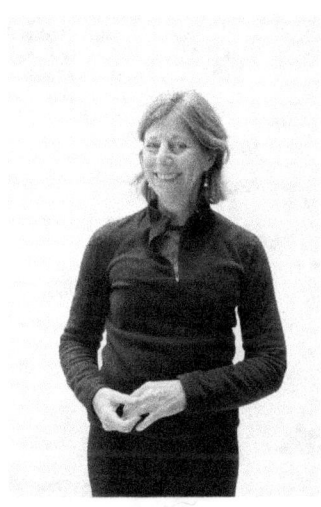

Whenever I have gotten onto a bumpy road on life's journey, I have drawn on the courage and openness that I learned giving birth. Fear can paralyze a person and block the true blessings awaiting them. During the time of River's birth, there was a movement back to natural ways of living. There were farm communes all over the country and people were driven by the desire to connect to the earth and sky.

Building one's life is a continual process. The joy of raising a child is manifest daily and the epitome is seeing a beautiful and successful adult, enjoying an adult relationship with him or her, and realizing that this is the flesh of my flesh and the bone of my bones.

The photographers of this book, Steve Walzer, and River's father Allen Cohen have both taken their journeys to the other shore. They were both loves in my life and they were also childhood friends. River's birth was a momentous experience for all of us, something that changed each of our lives forever. River was from the start, an amazing person, and still is.

Laurie Coe 2009

DEATH BIRTH LIFE

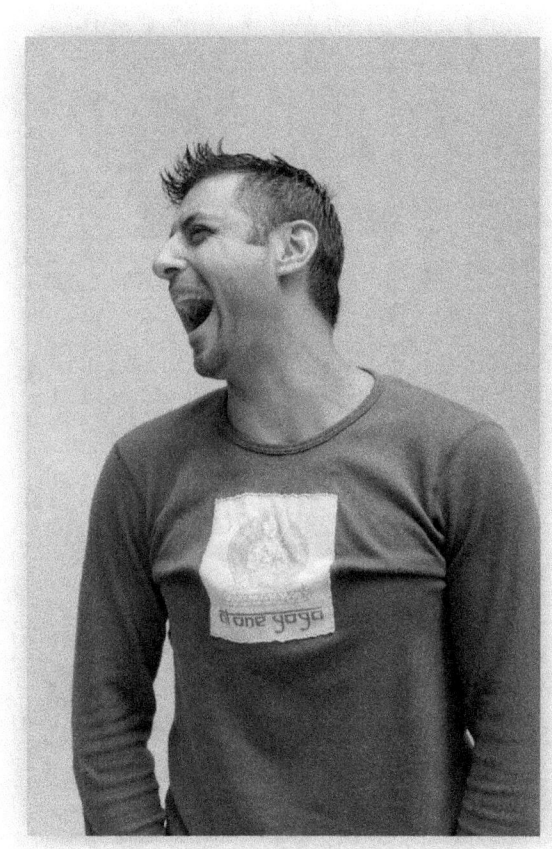

At this moment the wheel of life is accelerating and converging into collective consciousness providing a platform for oneness in the now more now than ever.

My Birth in Albion was a direct result of this convergence in the 60's with my father Allen Cohen as a primary founder of The Movement and the Aum family at Table Mountain was created with my birth. Laurie the sacred mother of my sister and brother lives now sharing love with all she meets. My life has evolved with these roots to one of complete awareness of these original concepts and the value they bring to our culture today. The death of Allen Cohen has created buds of life in a new generation within my own family and his legacy will birth a new movement of love shared between all beings.

It is with great appreciation and respect of Ann Cohen and all involved with the republishing of birth book, I hope that those who read and view these pages are brought new heightened awareness and change in perception regarding the cycle of life.

River Albion Elijah Cohen 2009

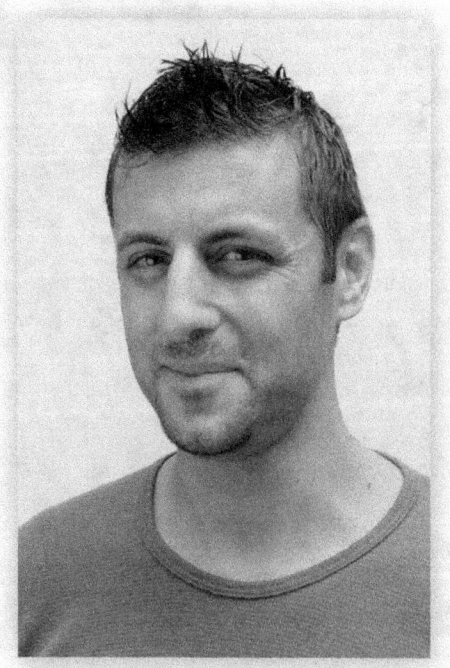

IV

Childbirth Is Ecstasy

Childbirth Is Ecstasy

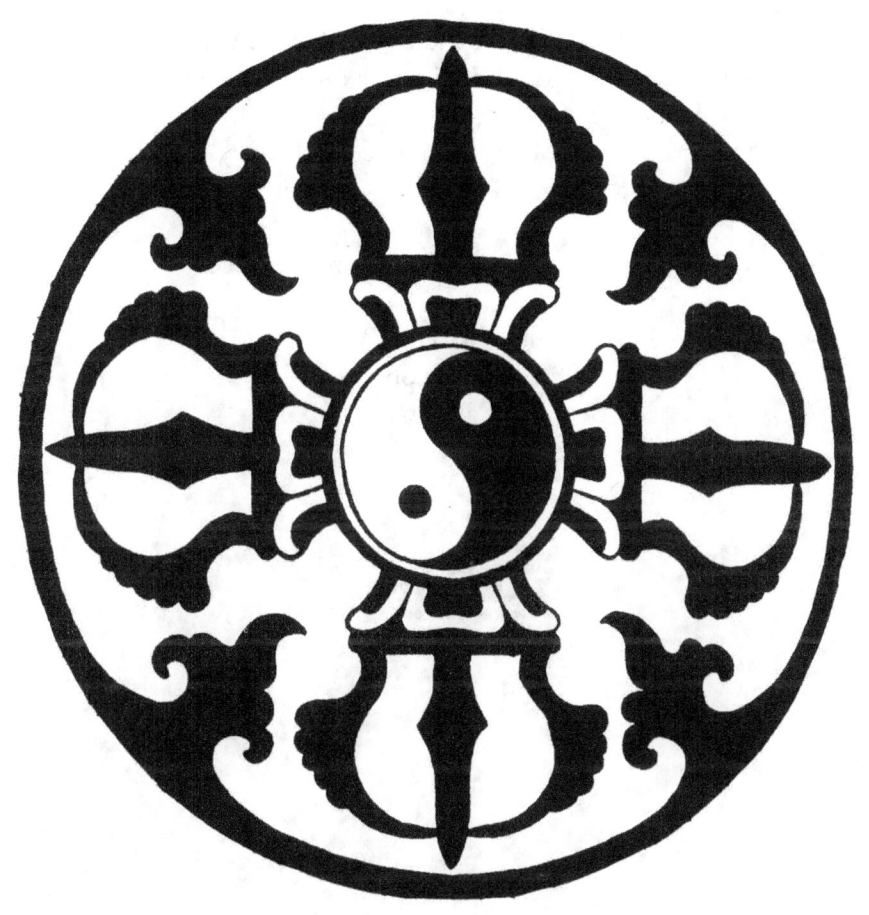

Photographs: Stephen Walzer   Word-Vision: Allen Cohen

Aquarius Publishing Co.

Front cover: silk screen rendition by Steven Walzer
of a relief statue of Mother Kali giving birth to the universe

Frontispiece: Tibetan Mandala rendered by Lama Govinda
for "Mandala" by Lama Govinda

Typography by Cranium Press, San Francisco

Distributed by Book People
2940 Seventh Street
Berkeley, California 94710

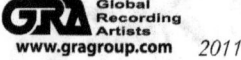

www.gragroup.com *2011*

Oh great Mother-Muse of the universe of generated forms

O courage beauty & love of human mothers

O perfection of the body-mandala through which we appear

*O compassion for sentient beings that will bring all to blissfull
fulfillment*

O to the 1 AM of a child's smile and sob and yours and mine

NOW & NOW & NOW

What new births
await the mind
of every moment's
Mary of beginning?

No more still
births of mind
But from the womb
of union will
The new christ of Love come.

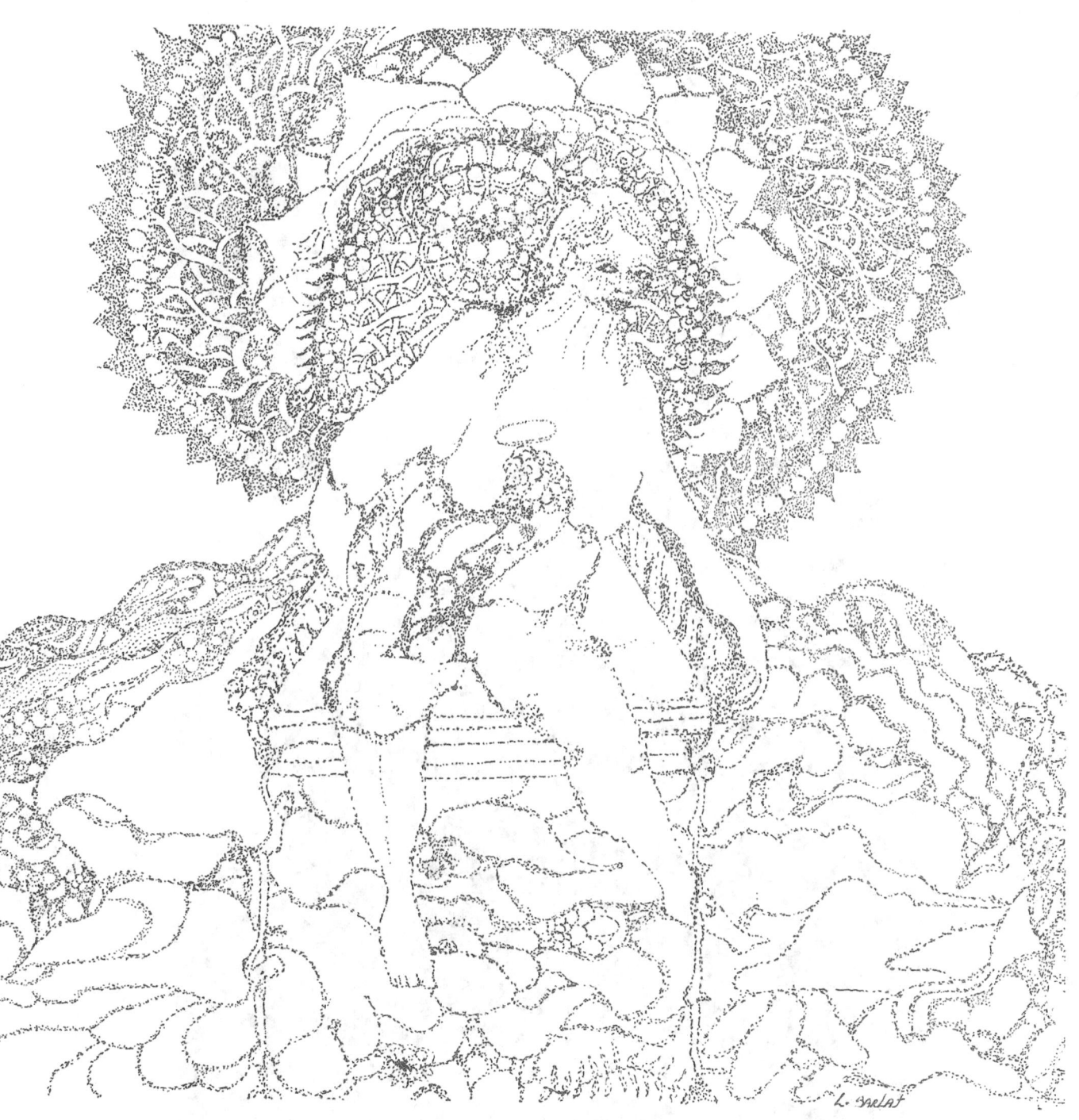

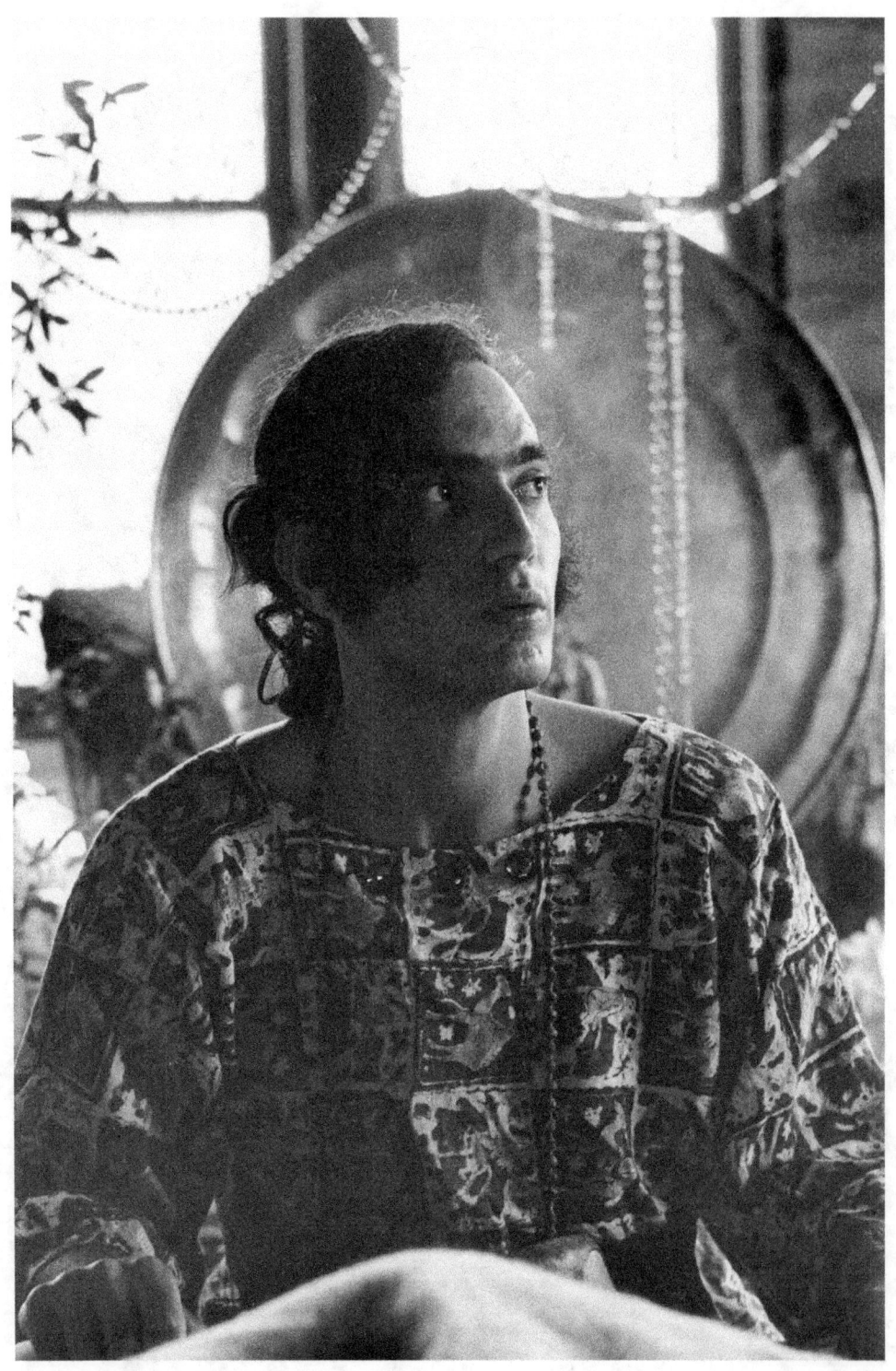

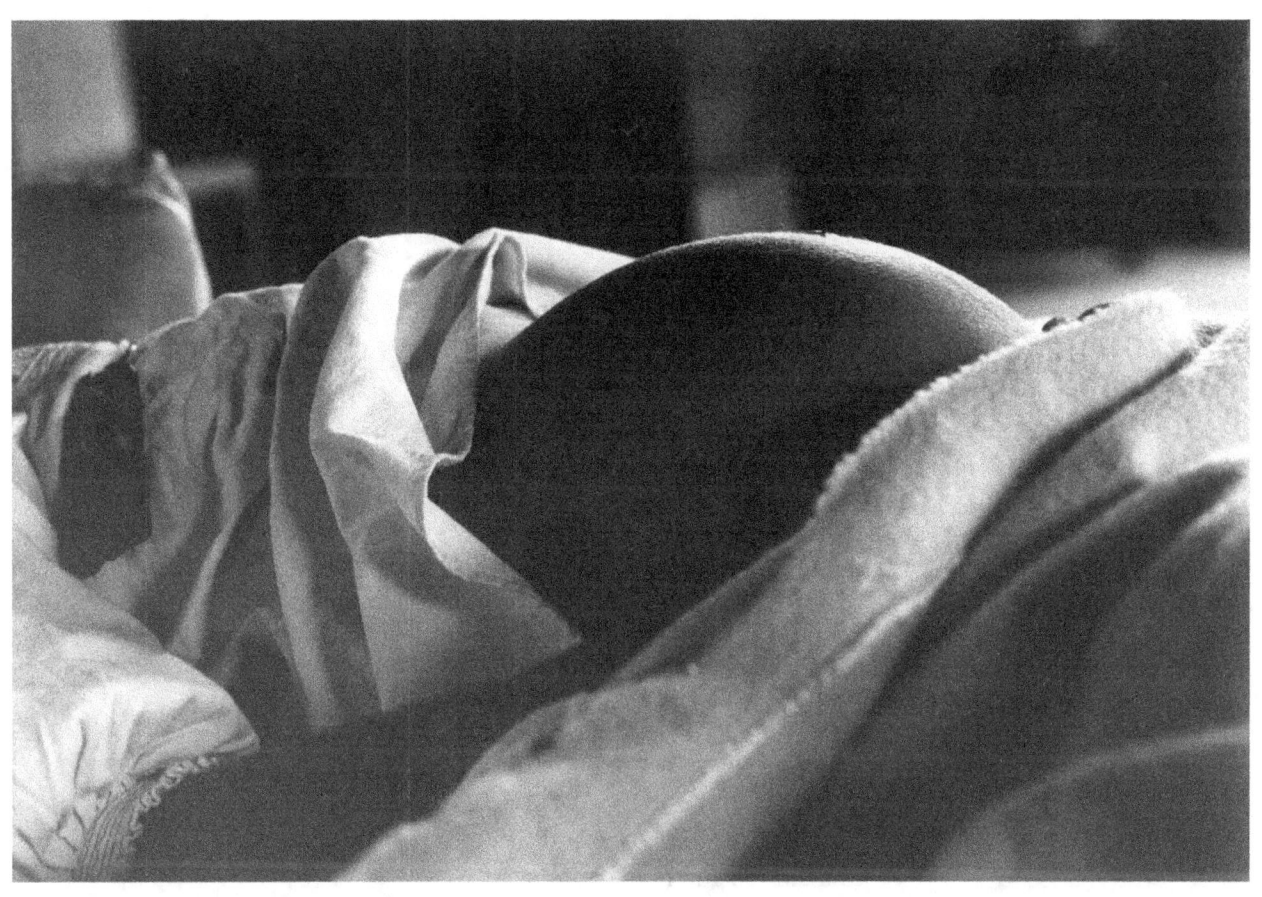

Childbirth Is Ecstasy

Rain drips from eaves
of newly designed and built house
in this communal settlement
of mystics and frontiersmen
Indians and ancient archetypes
incarnated in the midst of industrial age
rewed to the earth
on these hills of second growth redwood
fir, tan oak and pygmy forest;
land that looks like planet
when first vegetation and trees
arose straight and high
with primitive thrust
in the form of the spinal column
basic to evergreen, leaf and fish
to mammal and man.

This house part cook house
but designed dark and austere—
church stained glass with crosses
and other symbols shading
the grey dusk light strained through
the low fog glowing: dark redwood
boards and beams angle high
toward loft and tower.

Eight or ten men and women
stand and sit, lie, doze and pace
while Diane lies on her side

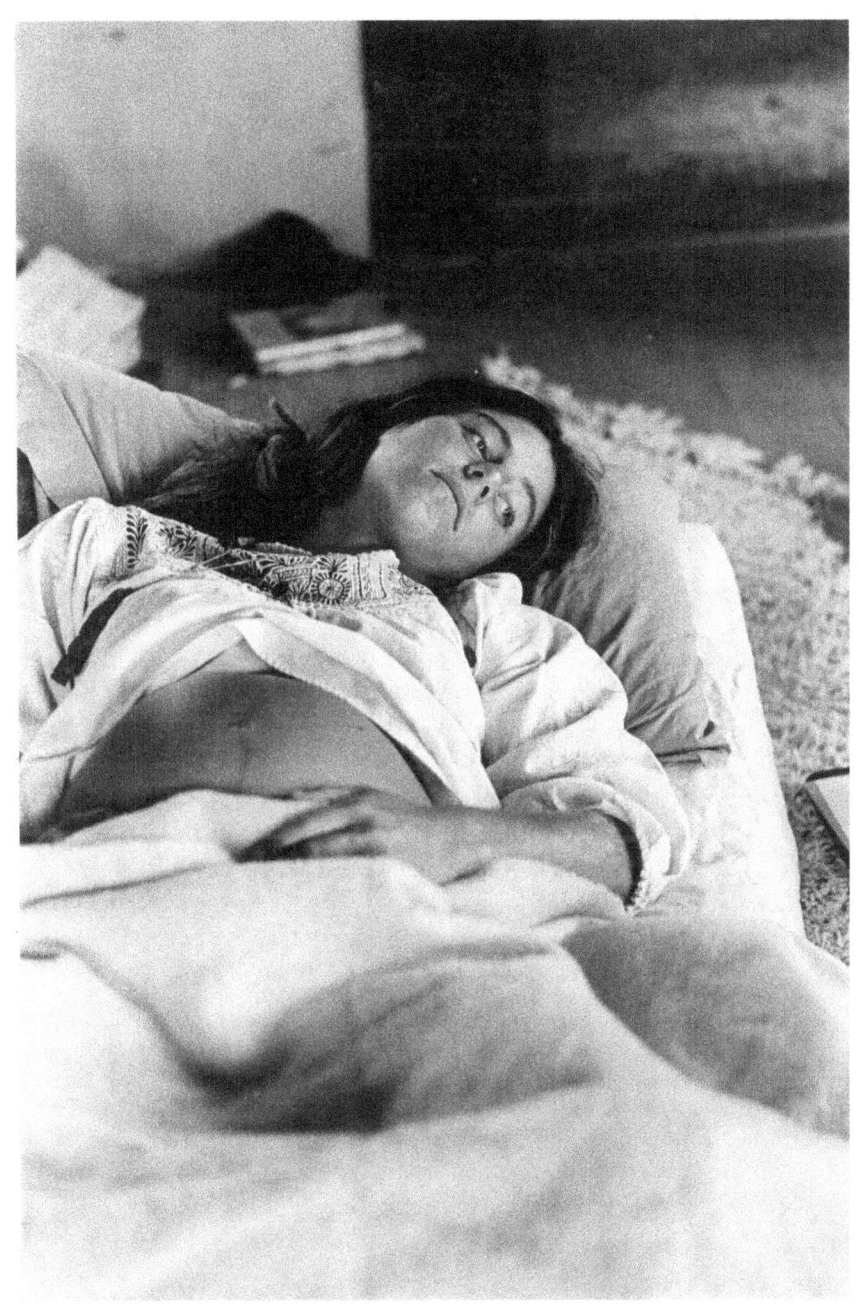

panting rhythmically and easily
in her 14th hour of childbirth;
fire burning in wood stove.
Her body huge breasted
prepared for milk of mother's love
dark and full, constant in her breathing
rooted, relaxed and aware.

Some of us chant;
Richard stokes fire
and plays dhamboura;
outside a drum beats
and occasionally a body cries
or speaks in questioning wonder.

Bill, her husband, at her side
whispering to her, caressing
and massaging her back
holding her legs, placing
wet sponge in her mouth
to quench her thirst—
preparing for months
to be part of act:
every day exercising
and breathing together—
now in one mind purposed
to be in com-union for
this new being's long journey
down a few inches of birth canal.

The rain lightly falls.
Diane pants and blows

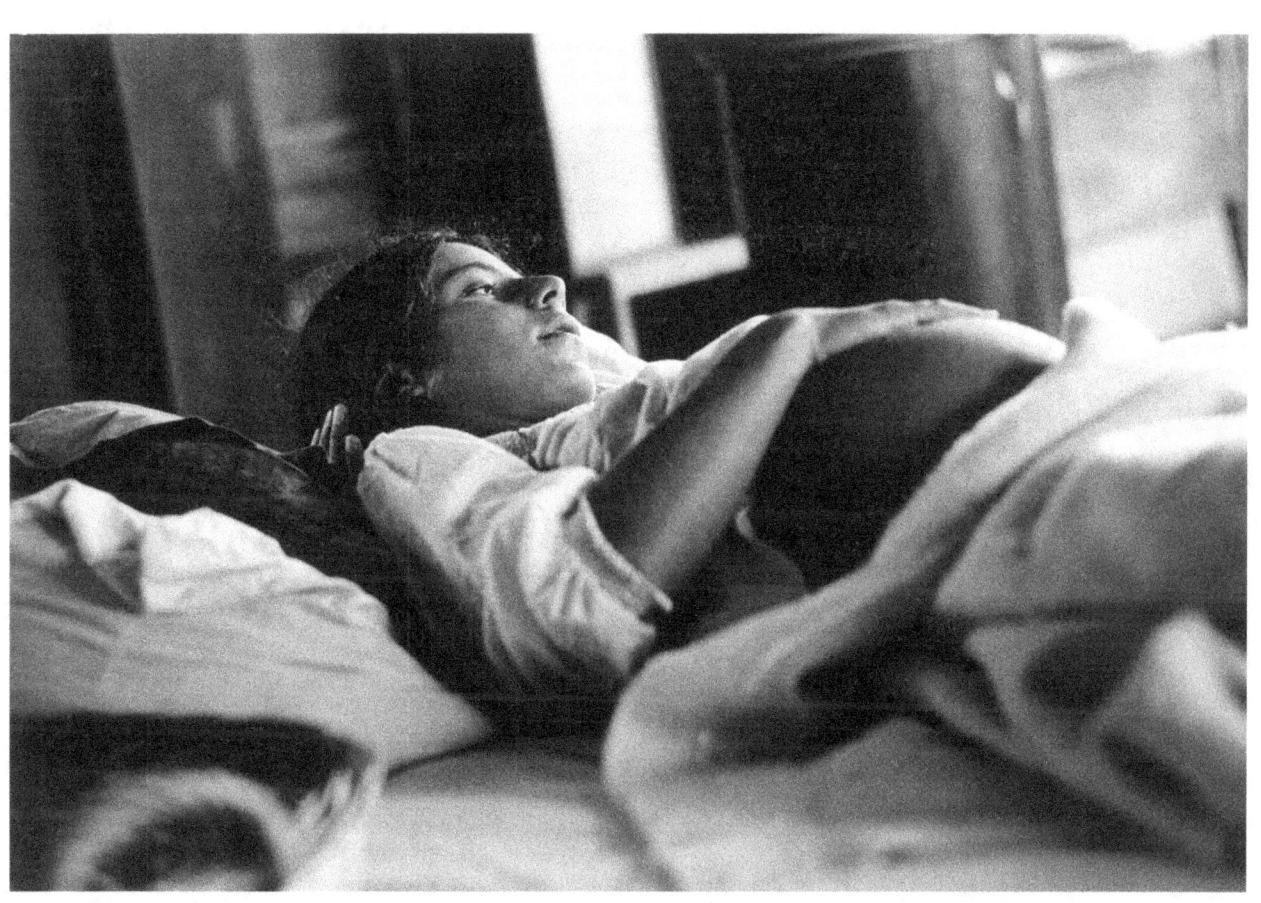

while we wander outside
in the late afternoon mist
to eat brown rice, carrots
and onions cooked over fire;
the grey mist timeless
hiding the sun's journey
over the ridges and valleys,
wind rippling in the trees--
waves rolling through Diane's body,
as this new being
already a week late
hesitates in its entrance
onto this planetary stage;
or perhaps Diane in a momentary act
mixed of embracing love and fear
won't release it from womb home
body grown nourished floating there.

Our family had twice witnessed
the act of birth and trusted
the perfection of nature--
Laurie and Vennie who were
conscious vehicles and actors
of these magic incarnations
breathing, chanting, praying
for these resurrections
toward evolution's veiled purpose.

Now watching themselves in Diane
in quiet confidence showing the way
forgotten rather than undiscovered
hidden by those who think birth
a disease and painful
debasing magnificent mothers
as pariahs and numbers
on an infinite sick bed
due to the mental distortion
originating in biblical
image of maligned EVE
leaving the Garden of UNITY
forever to manifest the floating world
in dire pain—Our ancestral Mother
whom the patriarchs of war blame
for breaking the harmony of the perfect plan—
Was that fruit of good and evil
the bearer of the idea
of self-generating egg
and free sexual activity
giving Mothers the power
of descent and immortality
inherent in the birth miracle?

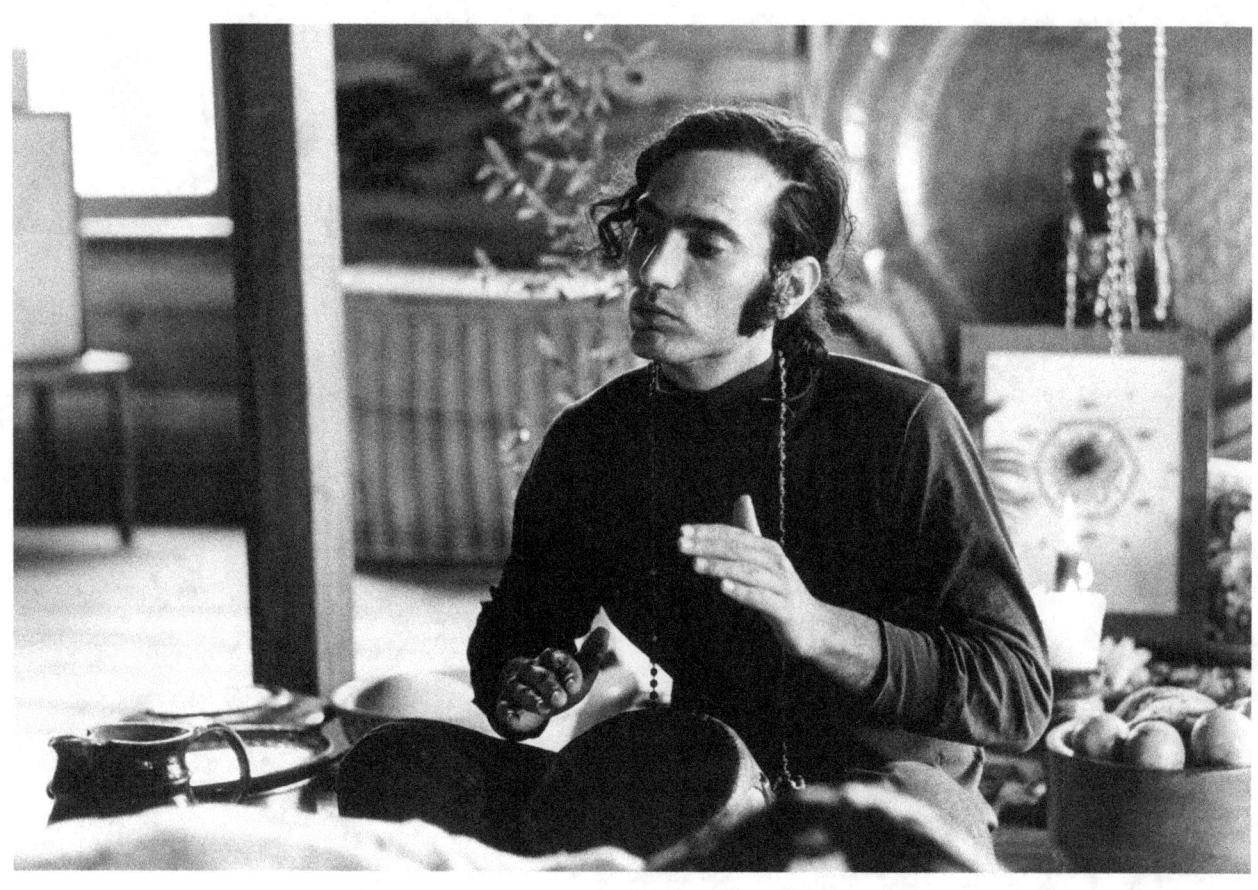

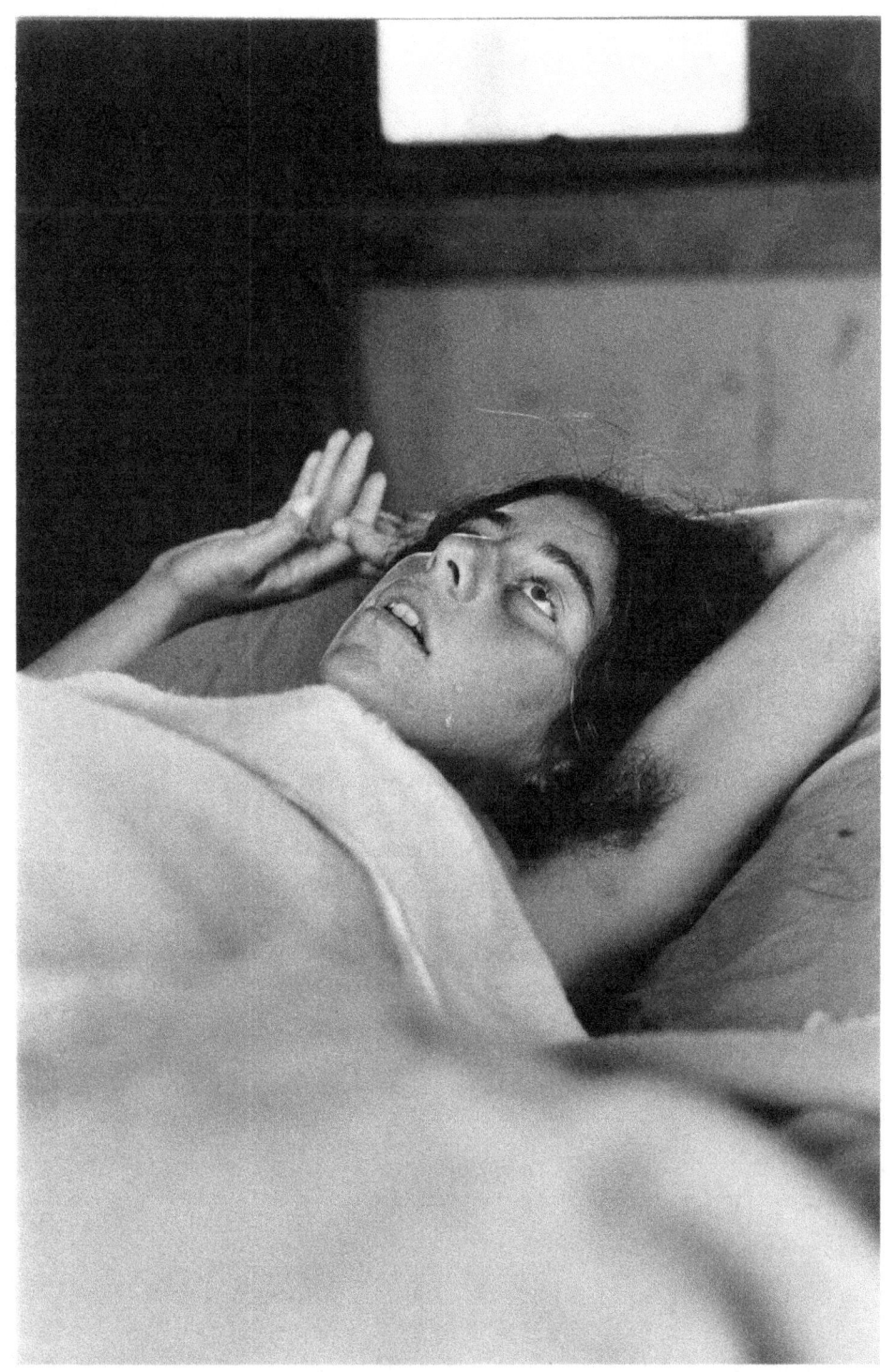

This biological power overthrown
by the hunter's brute power
based in the discovery of his cock and balls
as the carrier and deliverer of seed,
seizing matriarchal property,
extending psychic ownership over woman and child.
The hunter's power of blood sacrifice
and expanding wars maintained
thousands of years by cultures
of warriors and priestchraft;
the technology of war initiated
with the crossed swords
the fires of expulsion
and the murder of brothers—
These myths descended and guarded
by fearful priestcraft of doctors
with surgeries, analgesics and anaesthetics
in their fist:: the miracle veiled
behind a white sheet,
white linen puppetry of psychic
masculine war against
woman's natural ascendancy
hiding the revelatory,

the ennobling from her awareness
controlling the curtain of fear
by their dominance of technique
as if sentient beings have not
been born forever—
as 2 ½ year old Sanje
revealed this afternoon
"I can push a baby
out of my stomach;
I can push thing out of me."

I begin to see now the light
thru the dark cavern
of this age's mad war machine
and its urban laboratories
of greed conditioning:
thru a century of death's
screaming headlines
from Hearst to Huntley
causing hopeless bureaucracies
of rigid bodies, total solutions
and total weapons,
population suffocations
and senseless pollutions,
paranoia palace poisonings
extended to everyman's hut.

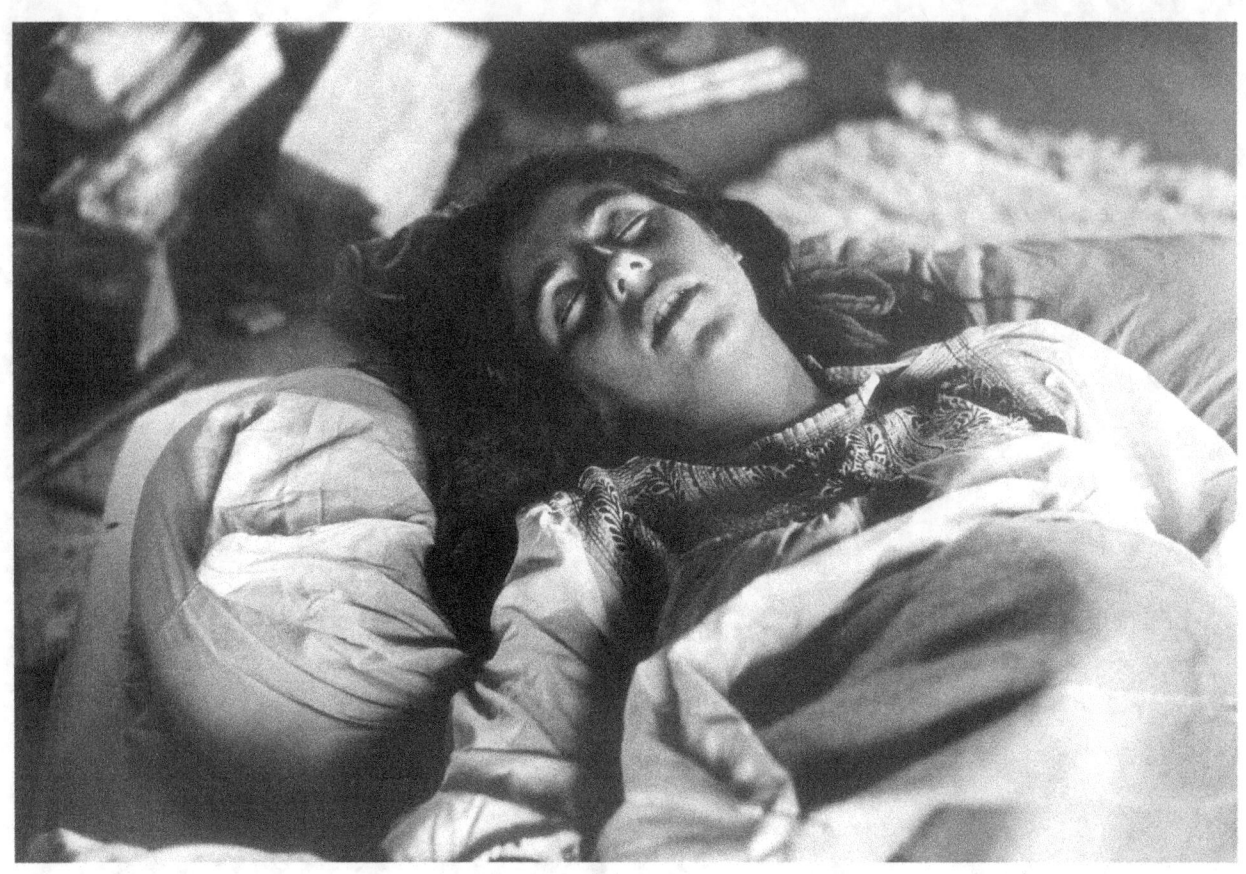

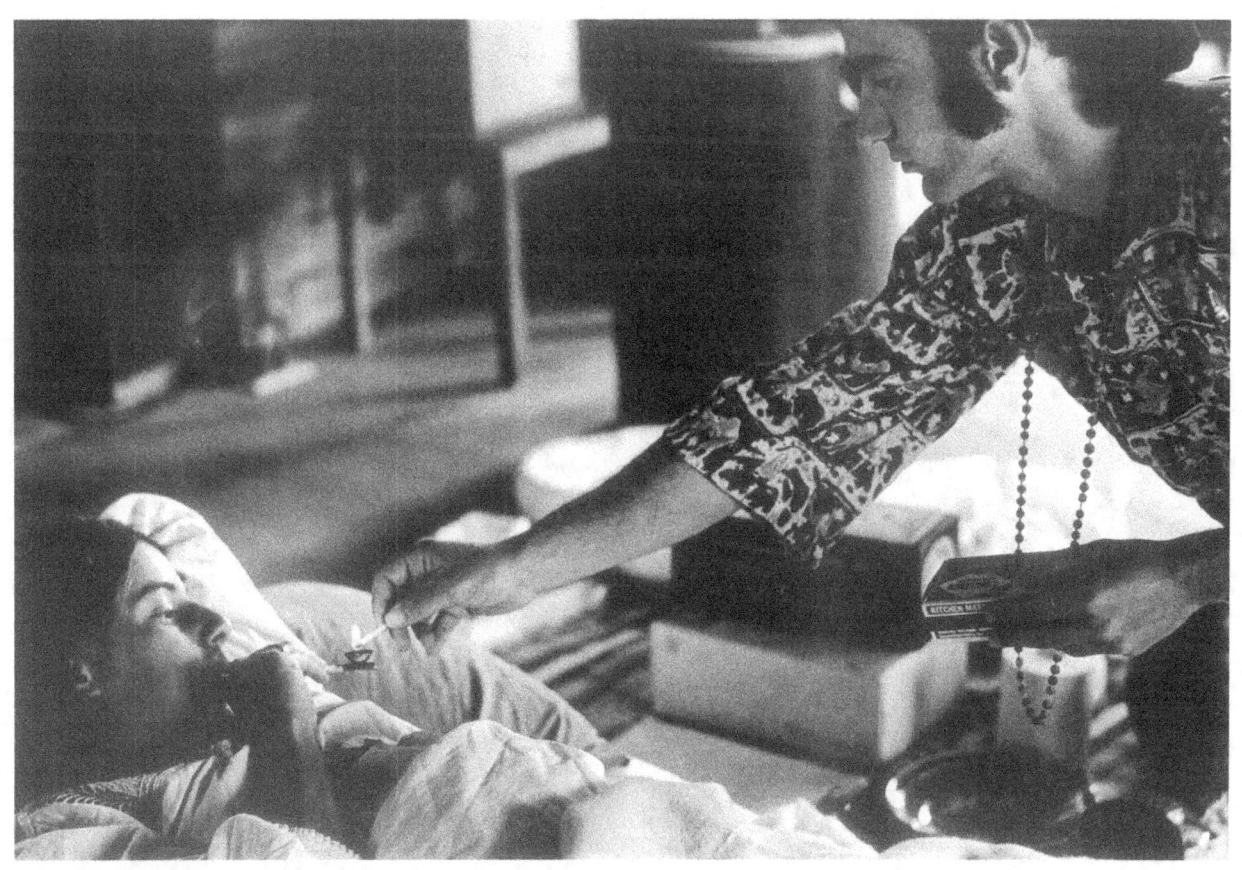

The light returns in life's natural rhythms:
in this act, this waiting
in the panting and blowing
in our pacing and sitting
as we drift towards 20 hours
of expectation with Bill whispering
in his wife's ear as a drum beat's
and dhamboura is strummed—
life's caring goes on:
dinner is prepared,
babies breast fed,
diapers changed,
wood chopped,
pant and blow
pant and blow.

The uterine contractions
(Walter says we should name them
bliss waves) come closer together.
Bill becoming impatient says
that he will call doctor
if child doesn't come soon.
Observing waves I say that
it looks like only an hour or two
until child comes home.
We all gather around the bed
and Pam and Bill give support
to Diane's tiring legs as
her panting becomes
more intense and longer
as length of waves increases
and period between waves decreases—
now child long wombed
leaves uterus and is
visible in birth canal.

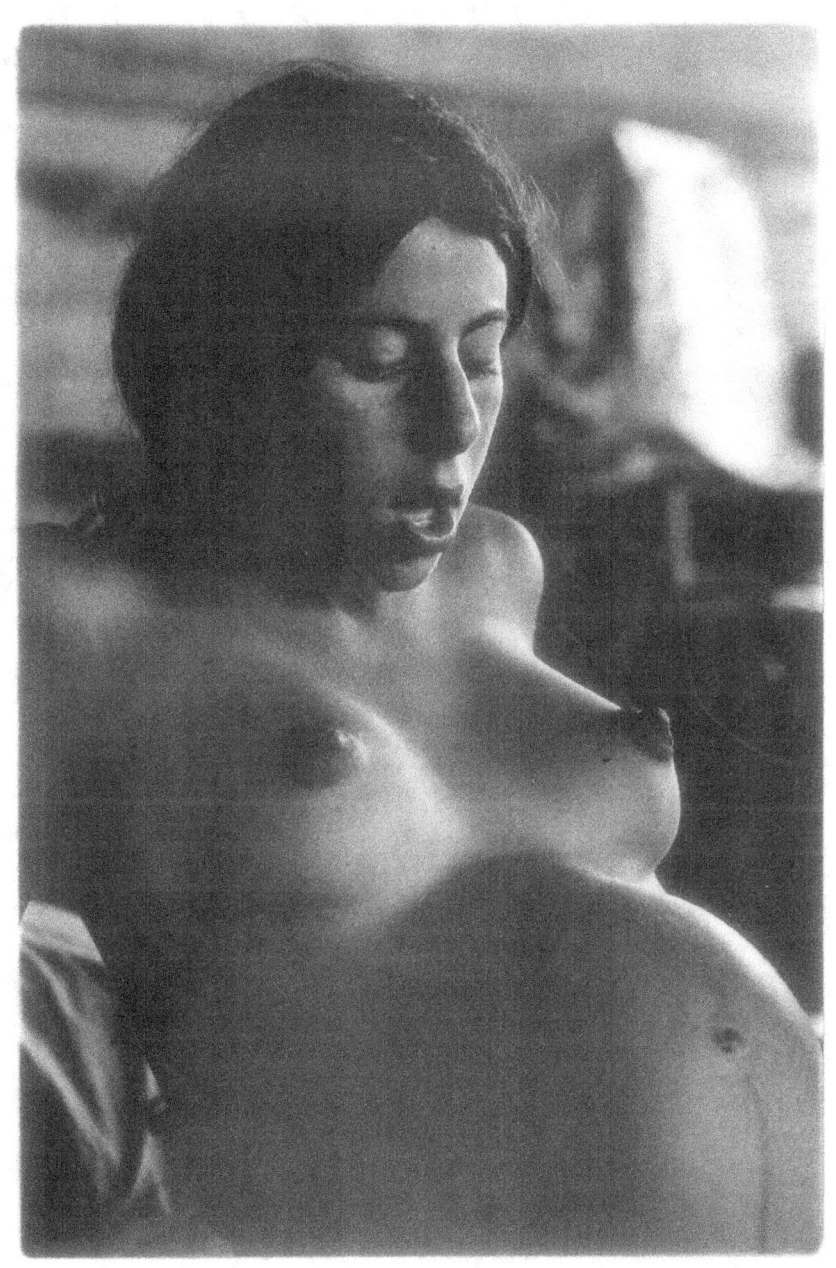

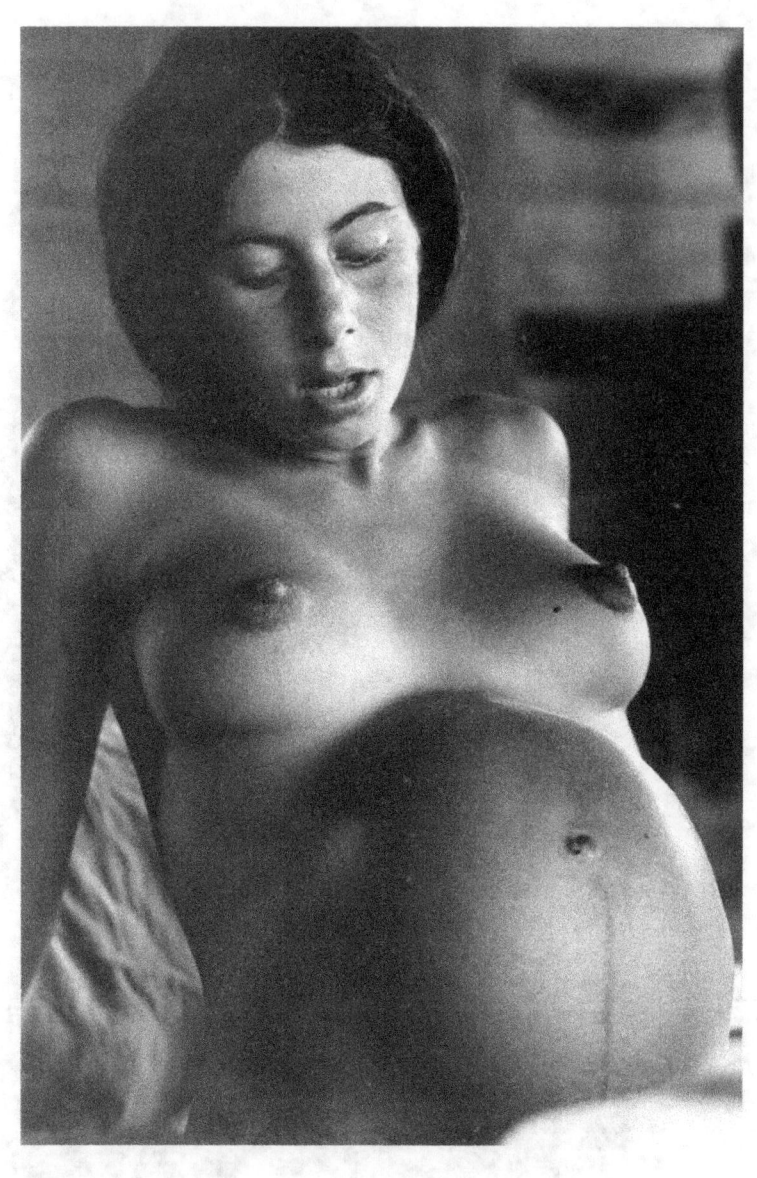

24

After washing our hands
with disinfectant soap
to protect against vaginal infection
I crouch between Diane's legs.

As I sit there waiting
I remember almost re-experience
the communion Laurie and I had—
the days lying on the meadow
learning the actual processes of childbirth;
breathing together estimating
the length and curve of waves,
chanting OM MANI PADME HUM
reabsorbing the lost intuition
of nature and wisdom of tribe—
here we faced and accepted all
the capacities of the universal Mother
whatever she would give we prepared
ourselves to take personally
and with full consciousness:
life or death or injury
to child or mother.
Heart to heart with the creation
we knew it was kind and good
only humans beclouded it with fear.

Before Laurie could fully practice
and perfect breathing patterns
child burst seal of womb
three weeks early and we prepared
quickly for sudden birth.
I called sympathetic doctor who
is more tribal shaman than M.D.
He told us child is fully formed
and grown and to continue with
our plans for home ceremony.
A few days later just before dawn
uterine water broke and
drained into brown September grass;
final signal for life's longest journey
from sea womb to atmospheric earth
the distance only a few inches—
blankets and Persian bag
full of frankincense, myrhh and hashish
in our arms, we walk slowly
toward communal ranch house
like tight rope walkers
along the curve of the earth
past redwoods, tan oaks and fir
and burnt out giant redwood columns
past wire fence and growing garden -
dirt road lit by candle
held in Laurie's land -
sea fog drifting along
ridges of the night.

House partly prepared for fireside
birth ceremony --- 12 people
waiting, apprehensive, hopeful;
for 3 months ready to participate
in veiled and feared birth passage.
Four women in this new tribe
with 7
children that came
out of their bodies
without their awareness
drugged, affeared, unfelt.
We enter large house
and sounds drift and awaken
everyone's lite expectant sleep
as Laurie bathes and
gives herself and enema.
Women awaken and become busy
with activity --- boiling water
preparing birth bed with
pre-boiled sheets and towels.
Men acting self-confident
and a little indifferent
drinking coffee and talking
about firewood for winter.
An altar is set up and finished
with pink Naked Ladies
from garden, fresh water
and a bowl of fruit; I place
frankincense, myth and hashish
in front of black Buddha.
I ask for gold and Walter
brings small gold cross
with "INRI" printed on it.
A visitor who had just shown
his paintings at Gallery of Mystic Arts
in Laguna places a drawing called
"Birth of a Child of Light" on altar
as a gift and an incantation—
showing a child with a bowl
on its head in the midst
of a field of flames—

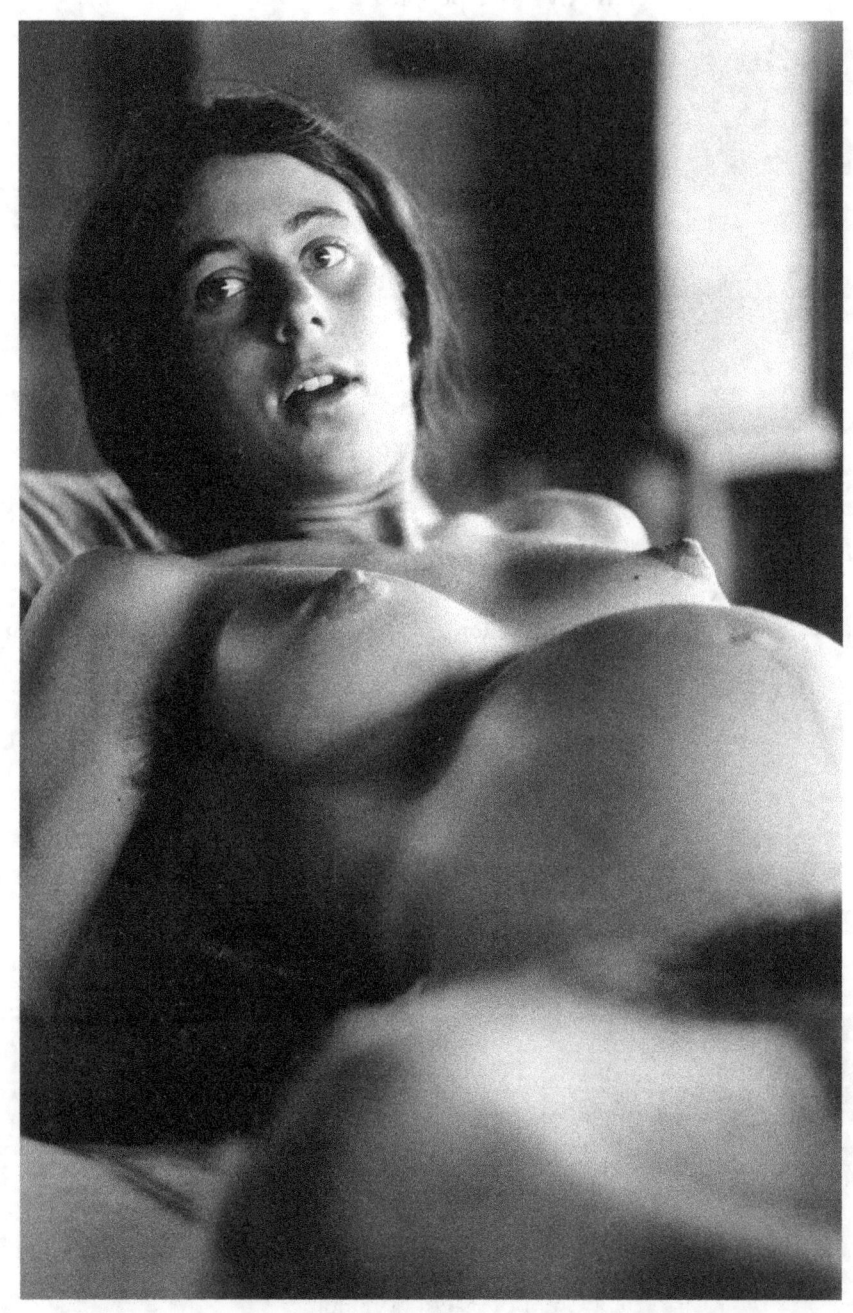

I mention that Buddha and Heracleitus
in India and in Greece
in the sixth century before Christ
said that everything was fire
and everchanging --- each moving
the world in seemingly opposite directions
with the fire of their acts and ideas.

Altar complete I shower and
put on clean ceremonial clothes.
Laurie gets comfortable on birth bed
and I sit down next to her—
for ten hours with fire burning
in fireplace she breathes and pants
and I chant and drum
light incense, smoke hashish,
breathe with Laurie's breathing
massage her lower back
put wet sponge into her dry mouth
and look into and swim
in her ecstatic eyes—
her breathing rhythmic and regular
and in later stage when waves
become intense she chants internally
OM MANI PADME HUM

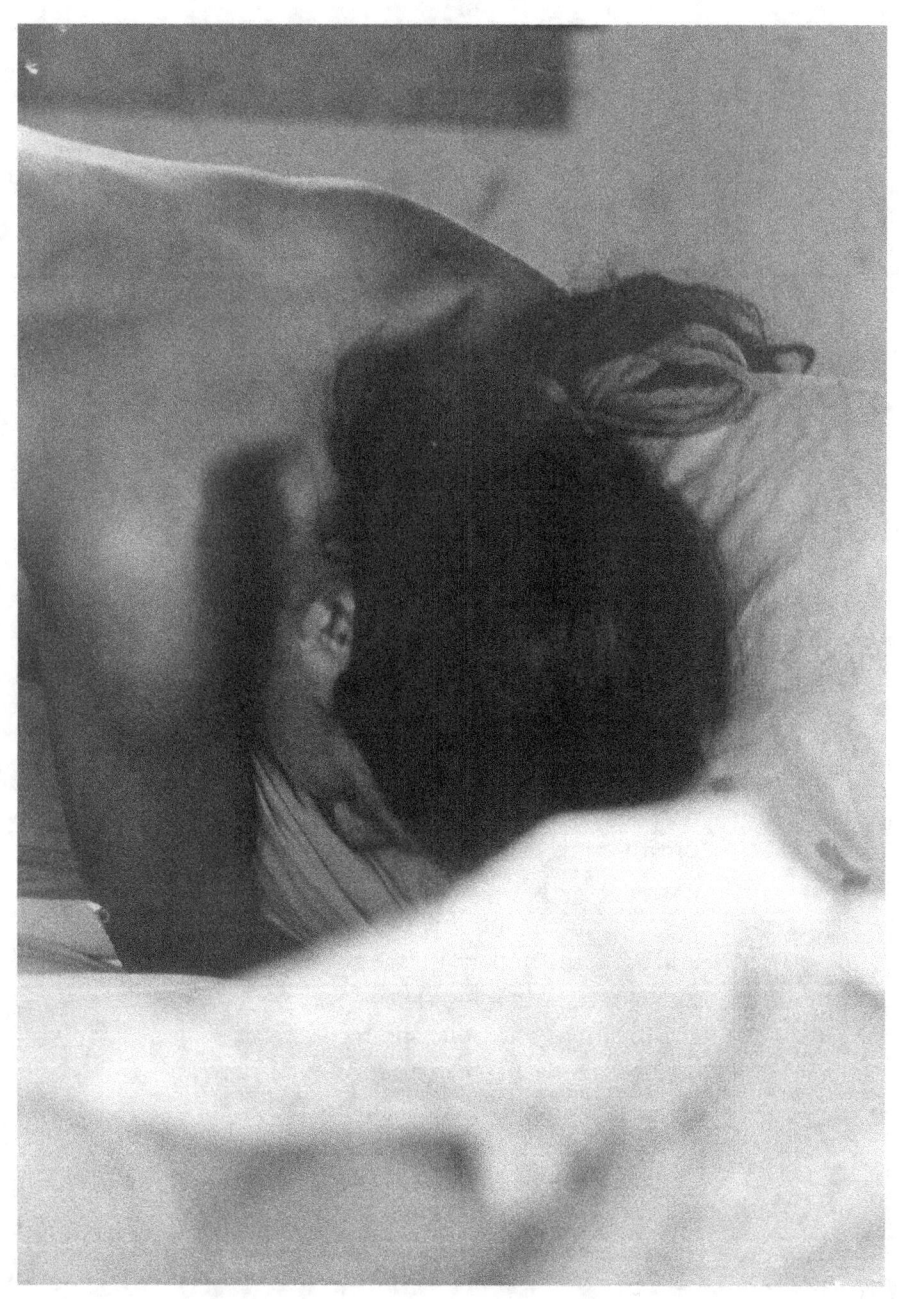

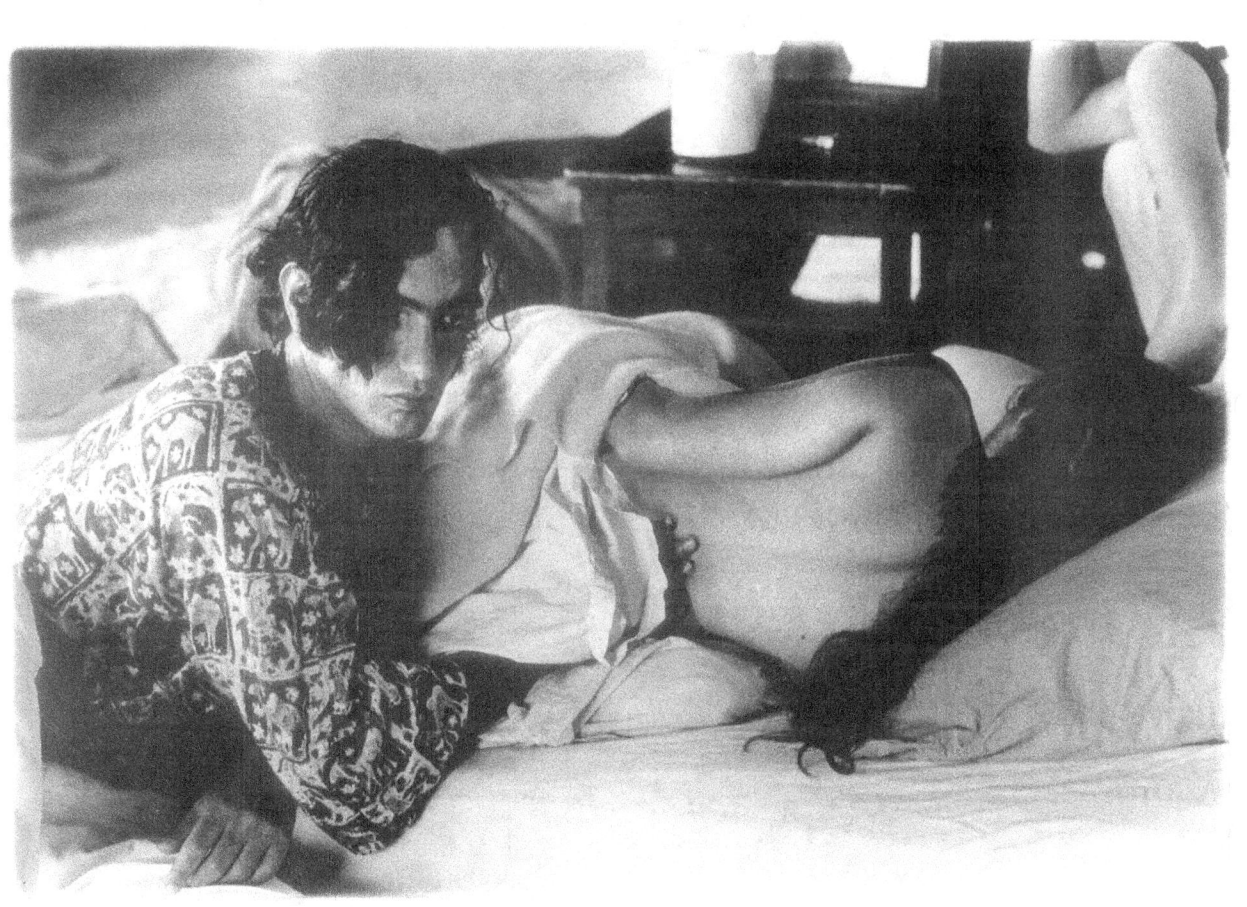

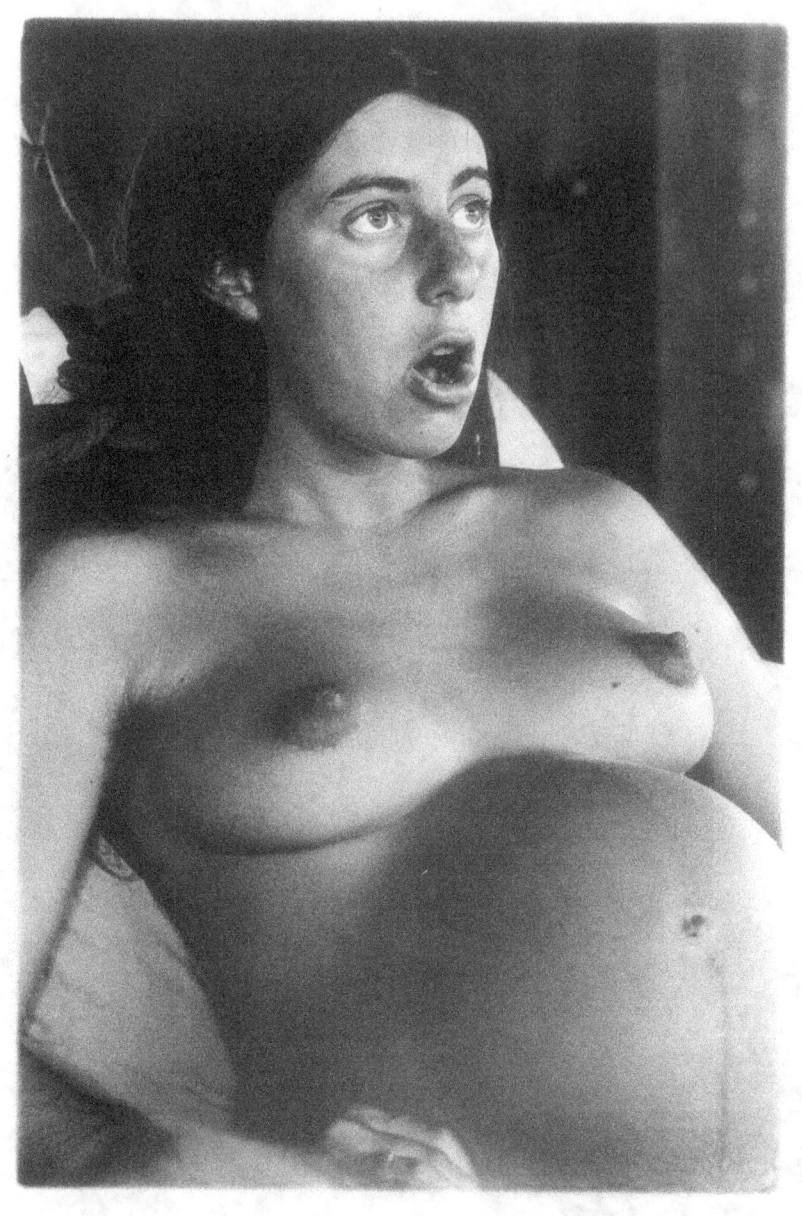

and I chant with her
as brothers and sisters come in
and go out sometimes chanting
or playing flutes or just watching
or bringing tea or supporting Laurie's legs.

At one point during overlong transition stage
while child is pushing through
cervix between womb and birth canal
she gets tense, loses her calm center
and gets up standing against a wall
for a wave and experiences another
on her hands and knees and one
on the porch with her hands
flung toward sun hazed over by fog
and one leg in the air dancing.
She returns to bed and Pat
who birthed two girls helps her
to relax and breathe with waves again—
all this time I feel united
yet distant from the
immaculateness of the internal
and alone experience
fusing Laurie to this creation,
except to be there and be calm
and have a strong faith.
At the tenth hour Laurie again
panting and breathing regularly;
some of us chanting and drumming—
she says she feels like pushing.

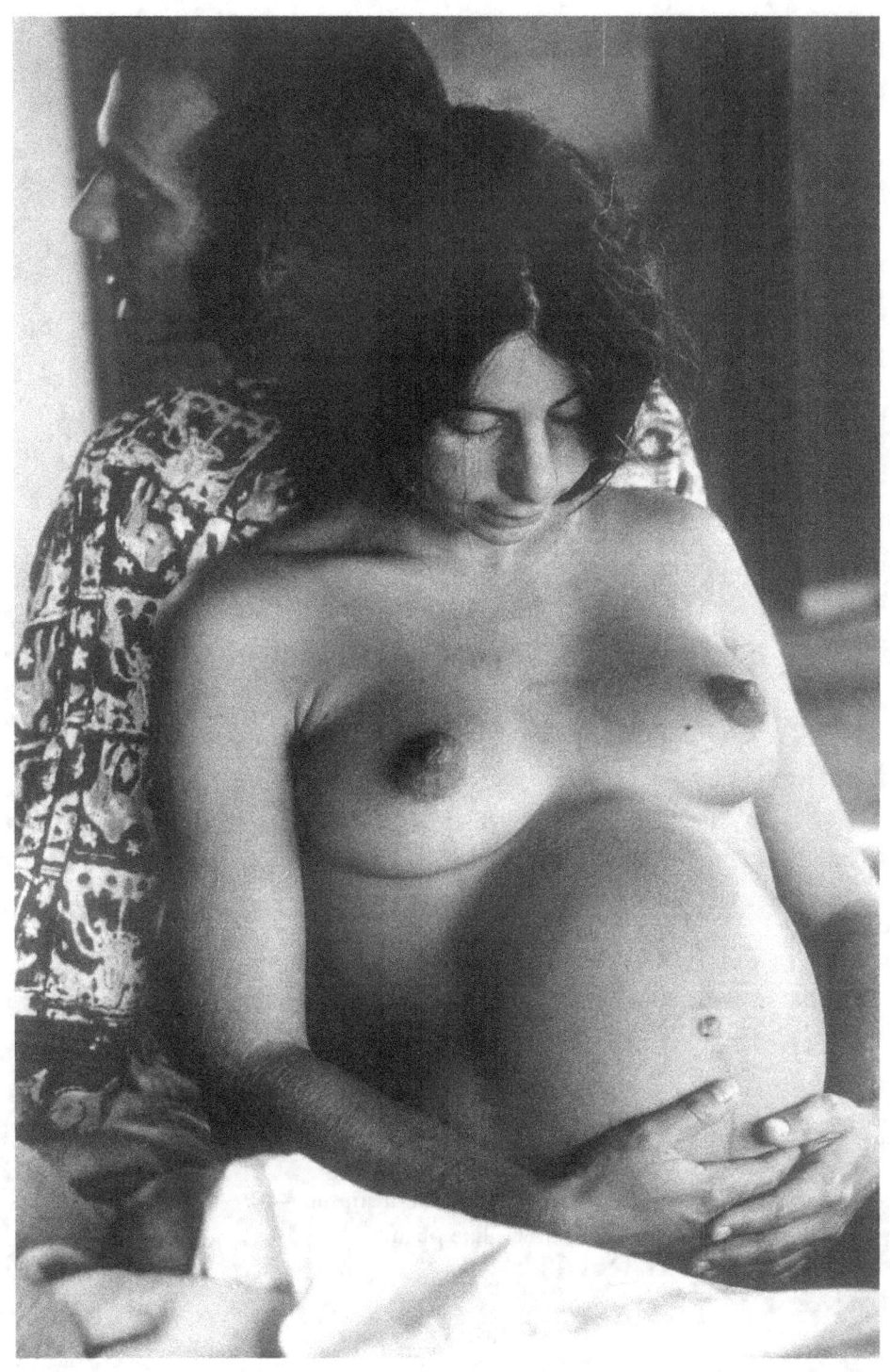

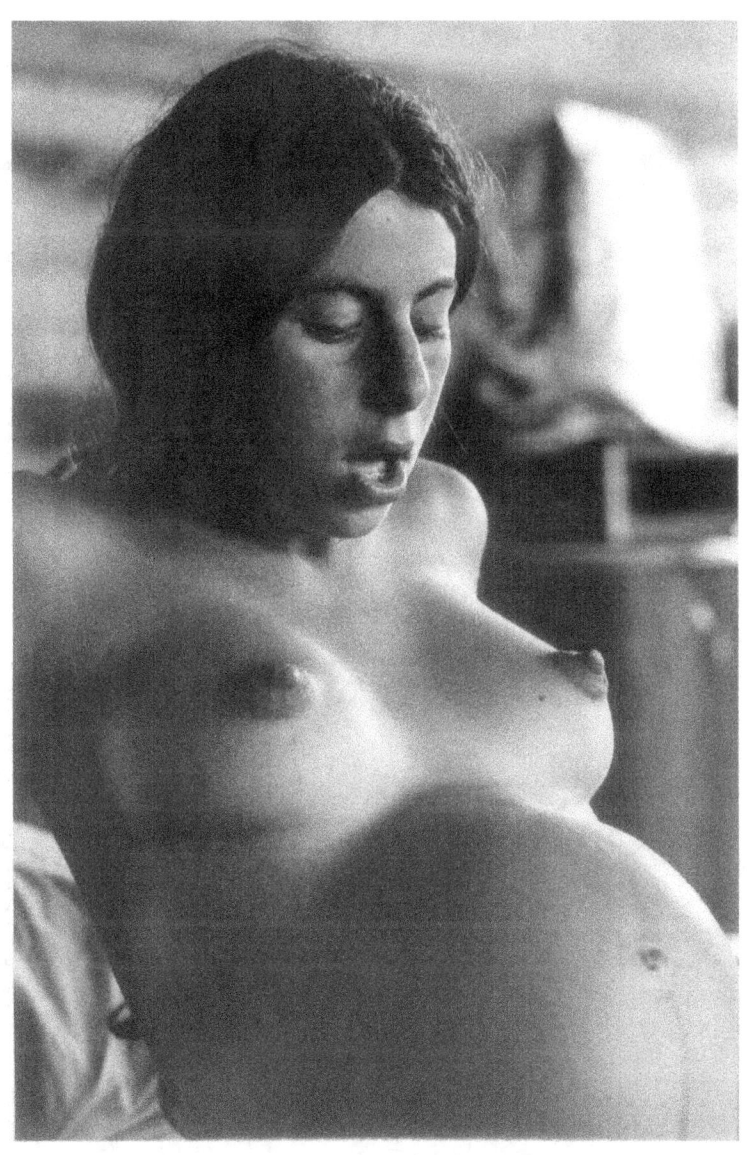

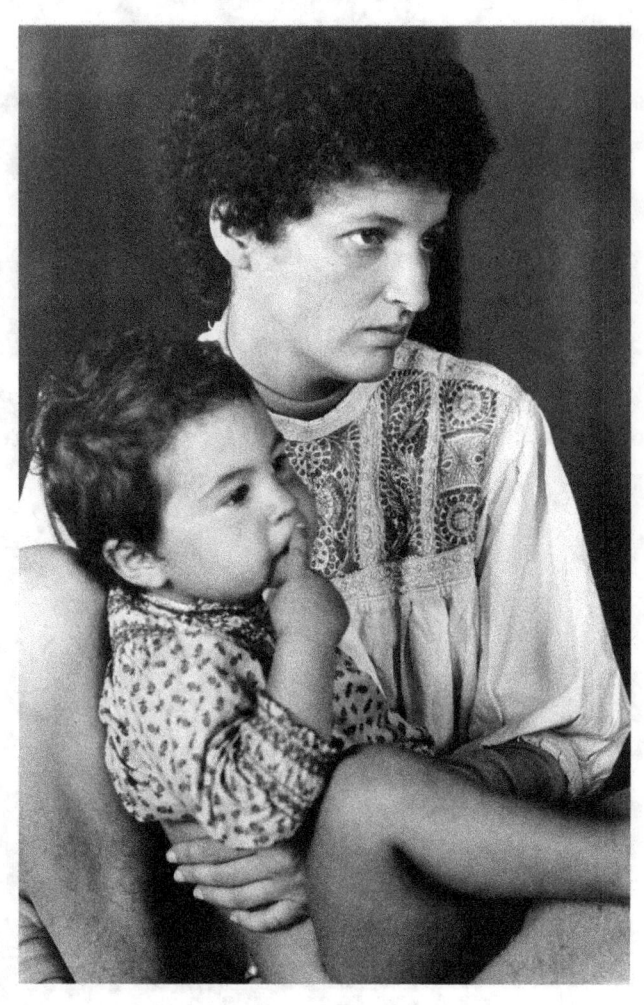

We look deep into her yonni
and see a black shadow—
we know the child is coming
the cervix finally open and traversed
and a new person in a body
inspired with the soul desire
to be world-born
is rocketing toward us.
We raise Laurie on the pillows
and now she pushes and breathes
with inner determination and strength
to aid child's passage down canal;
we all gather together now
chanting OM MANI PADME HUM
with deep intensity—
Bill Bowen and I wash hands thoroughly
with boiled water and disinfectant soap
to prevent internal infection in the mother
and I crouch between Laurie's legs:
clean bed pads are placed
on bed by the women.
With each push the dark shadow
moves closer to us—
Laurie's aura is a deep violet
of sunset in redwood valleys.

Bill who was only man in Mendocino area
who had participated in and experienced
his wife's childbirth and maintained

piercing the ocean of the unknown
and forgotten separating us from
this natural beauty emerging from dark womb
to sunlight --- the drone of the chant
and Laurie's breathing and moans
as she pushes sounding an ancient harmony.

As I crouch between Diane's legs
this moment and my mind's recreation
of our child's birth merge into one act
I extend my hands while Bill Chase,
Dian's husband holds her legs and arms
for support as she pushes just a few times
and a bald head appears
at mouth of vagina
a white pulsing vein at its top.
I tell her to stop pushing
to allow the uterus to do
the rest of the pushing itself;
but next wave doesn't advance
head too much so she decides
to push again and then its angel head
covered with white lace membrane
spotted with vermillion blood nutrient
throbs in my palms light and human faced
and next wave ejects body
from womb to planet
]a perfect design of male human
spontaneously breathing
with its first cry—
a new voice on earth—
we remove excess mucous and fluids

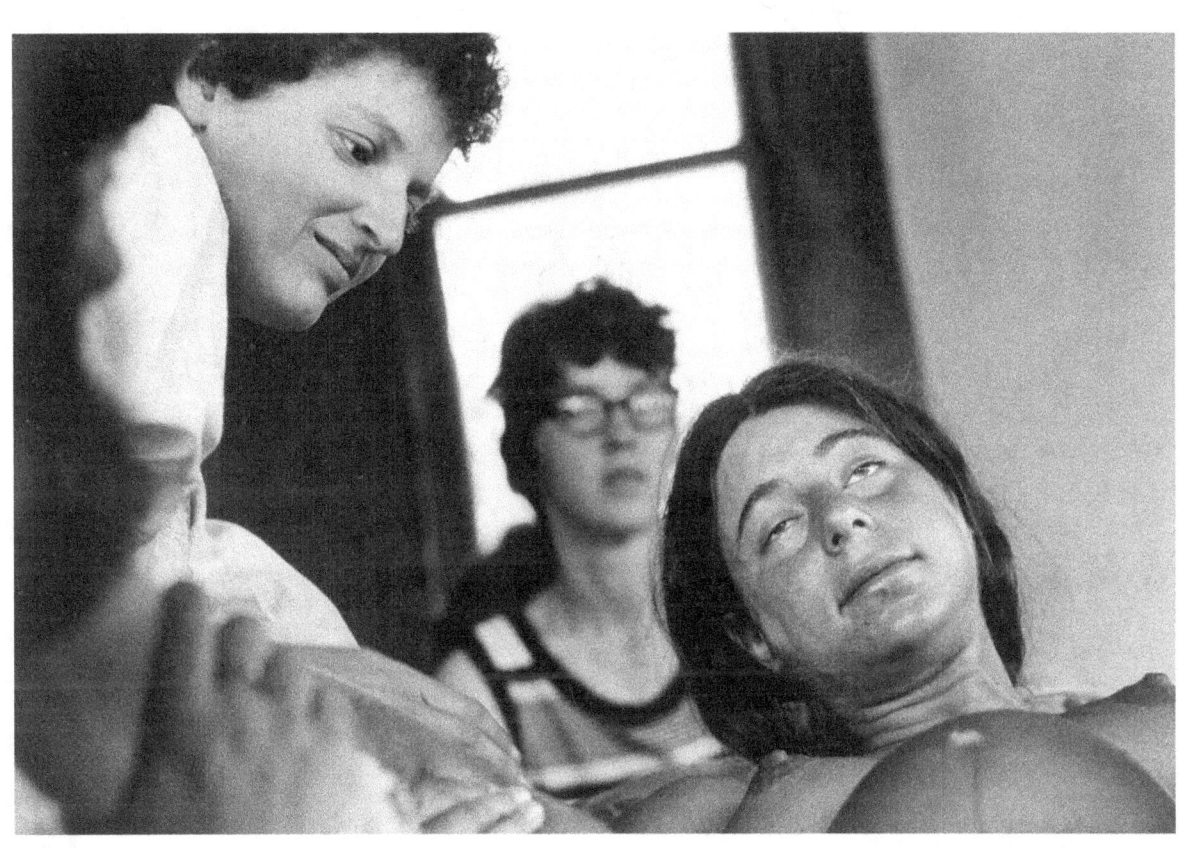

immediately from mouth and nostrils
with sterilized rubber aspirators.
I hand male child to Diane
she receives him glowing
and lays him face down on her belly
while all the women cry with the happiness
of witnessing the complete miracle of birth.

After 15 minutes of group admiration and joy
I take umbilical cord still attached
to womb-life sac inside Diane
and mild remaining nutrients in cord
toward baby now sucking at Diane's
huge but still milkless breast—
(milk sometimes takes 2 or 3 days and
on rare occasions up to five days to come in)
I take blue color-fast ribbon
(though white shoelaces would have been better)
and tie a tight square know
about half way up the umbilical cord;
then with another ribbon I tie
a second square knot about 2 inches
from baby's belly and cut cord
with sterilized scissor about ¾ inch
above this knot and he is free
individualized male being.
Soon there is another wave
and placenta—9month womb home
and nourisher of life is expelled
from body—its work done.
Bill says he will feed it
to his beloved dog.
Everyone happy and tired

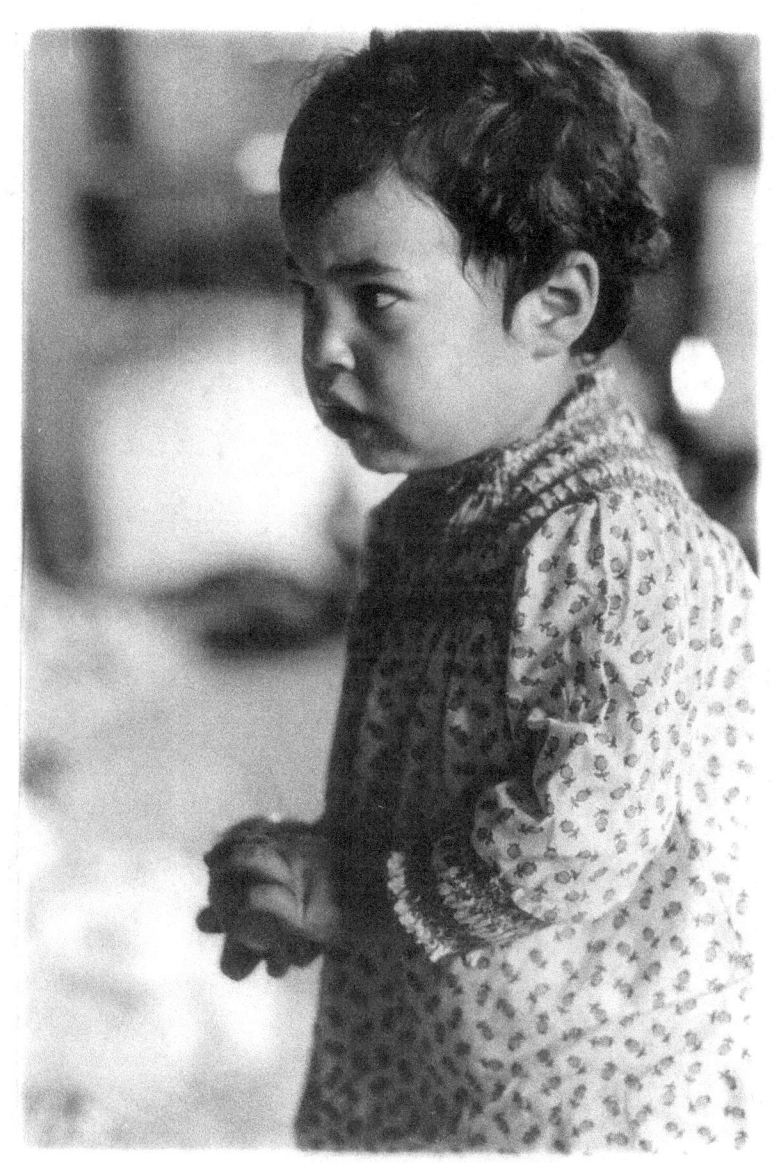

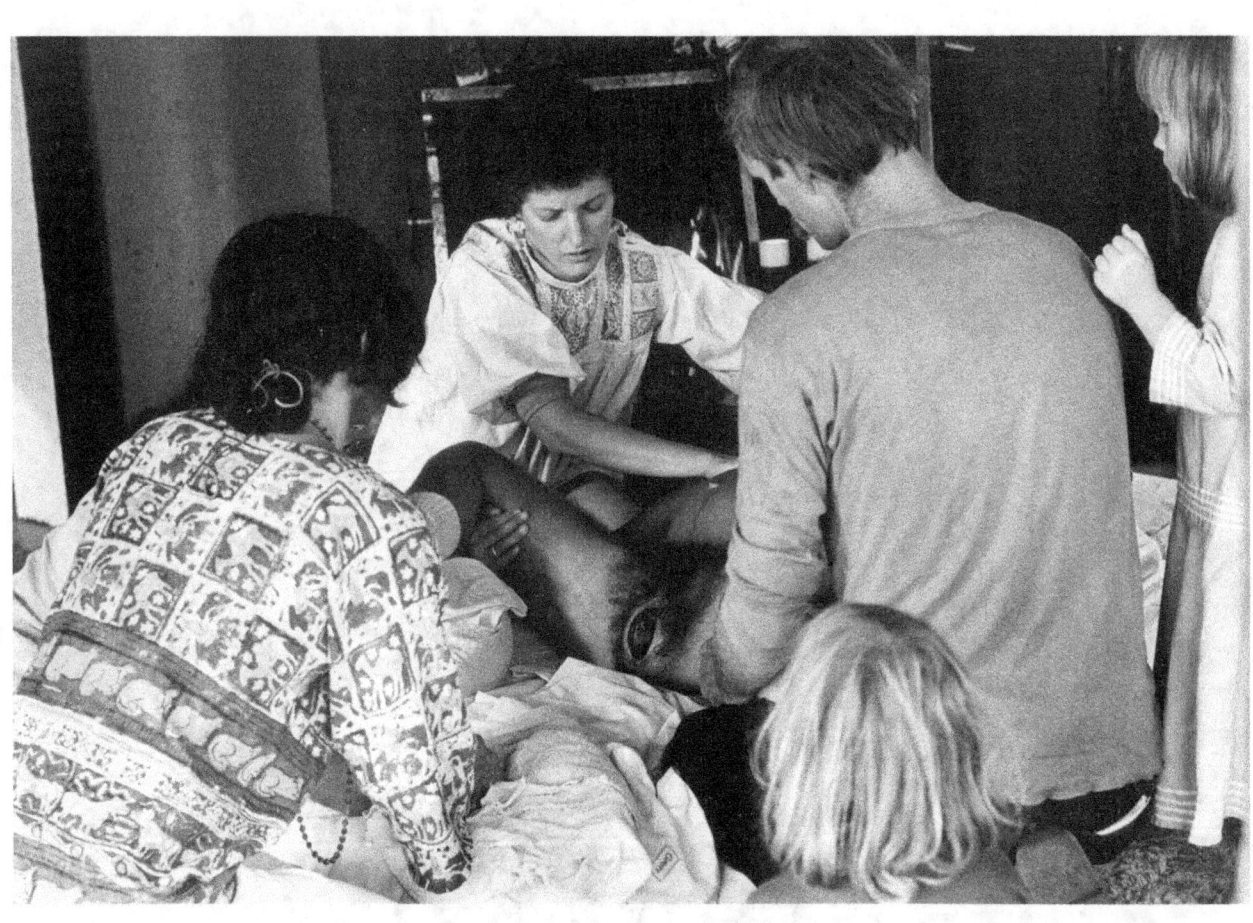

I think again of our son's birth.
Though it was a shorter labor
how strange and difficult it was
he was in depths of birth canal
for about 20 minutes with Laurie
pushing heart and soul and 10 people
chanting OH MANI PADME HUM.
Finally a silken hairy head
appears at mouth of vagina;
I stretch my hands out while
Pam and Bill support Laurie's legs—
my palm are up and I wait.
Bill says, "Let's sing a Hebrew chant."
And I begin chanting
"SHMA YISRAEL ADONAI ELOHEYNU
ADONAI ECHOD" (meaning
"Hear, O Israel, the Lord our God,
the Lord is One:) and the dark head
comes out a little further with
wave and push and then recedes
a little in moments between waves.
(We didn't remember to advise her
to stop pushing when head crowned.)
Her Yonni stretches wider and wider
as the black haired head emerges and fills it—

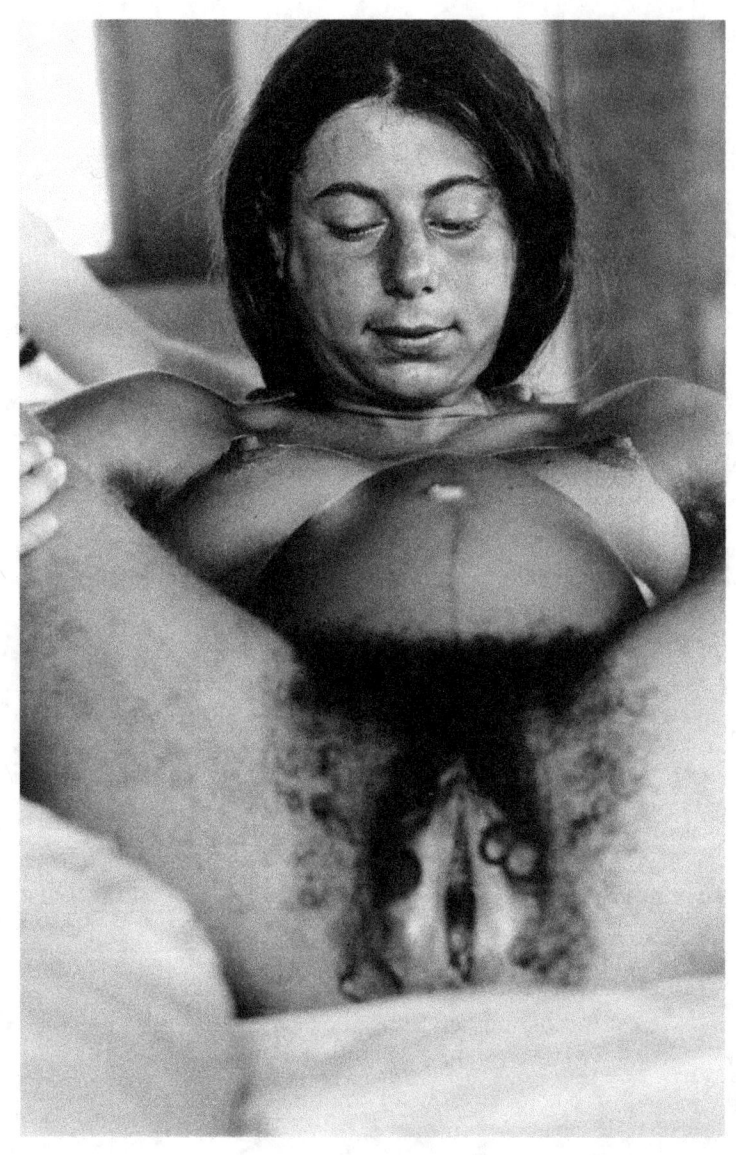

44

this coming and receding goes on
for about 15 minutes, much longer
than it ordinarily does, but
Bill reassures us "It's all natural,
each in its unique way,
just relax and keep up your breathing."
We chant and watch and wait.
As the head bulges in vaginal mouth
we watch the perineum
the skin between vagina and anus
slowly rip open and blood
drip from its edges.
We look at Bill wondering
if something should be done.
He says, "Don't worry it's a minor
tear look at the beauty being born."
Laurie continues to push
and to relax between waves—
her color turning scarlet,
her strength and will everlasting
more beautiful than any Venus.

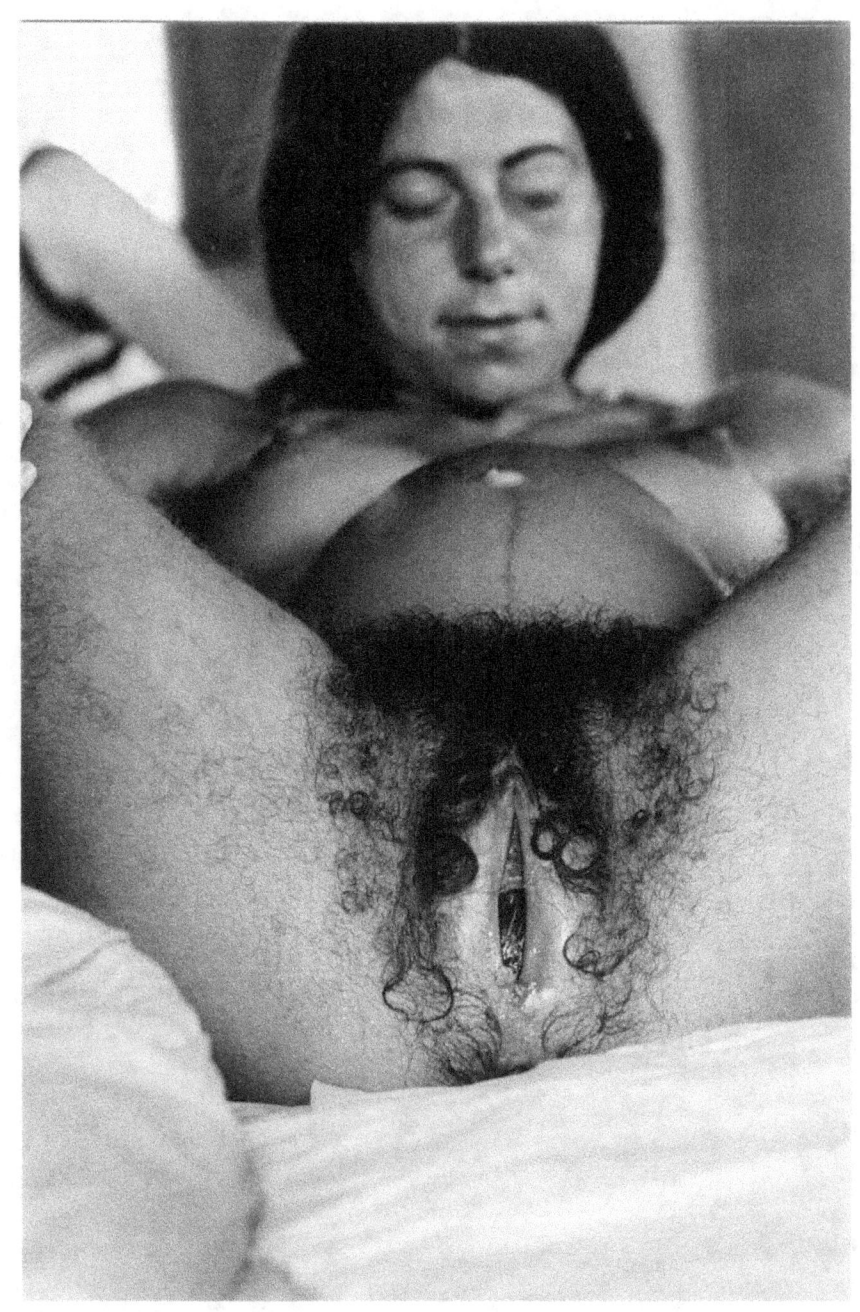

46

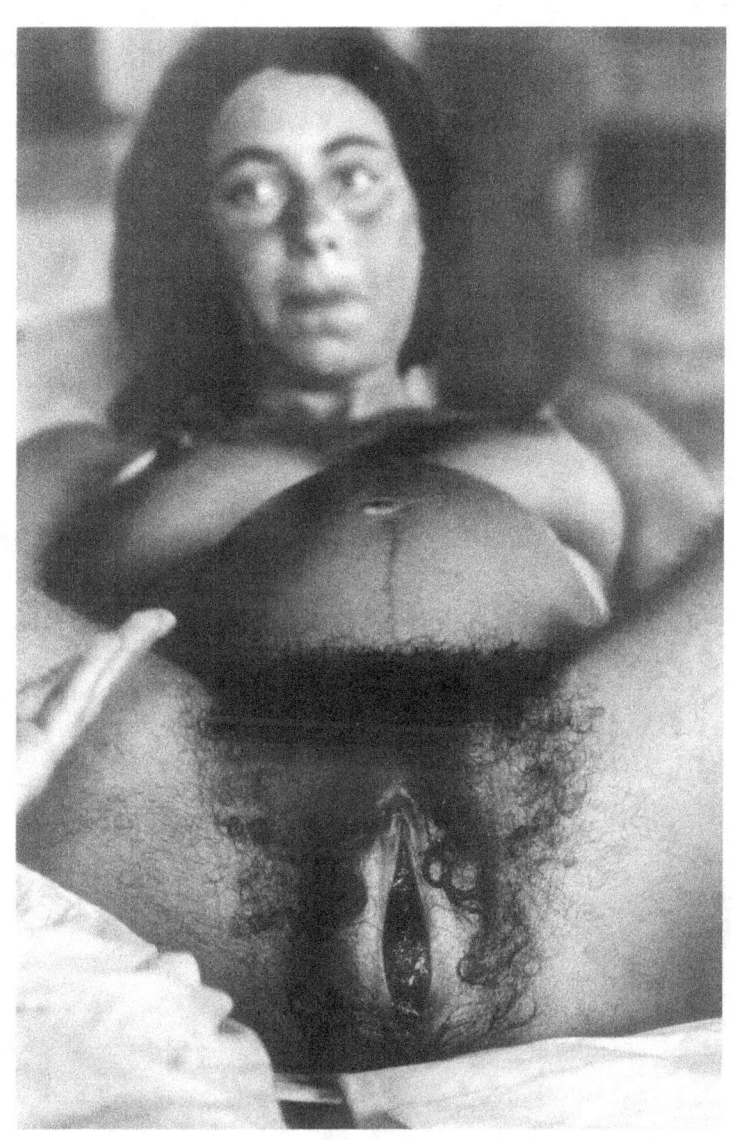

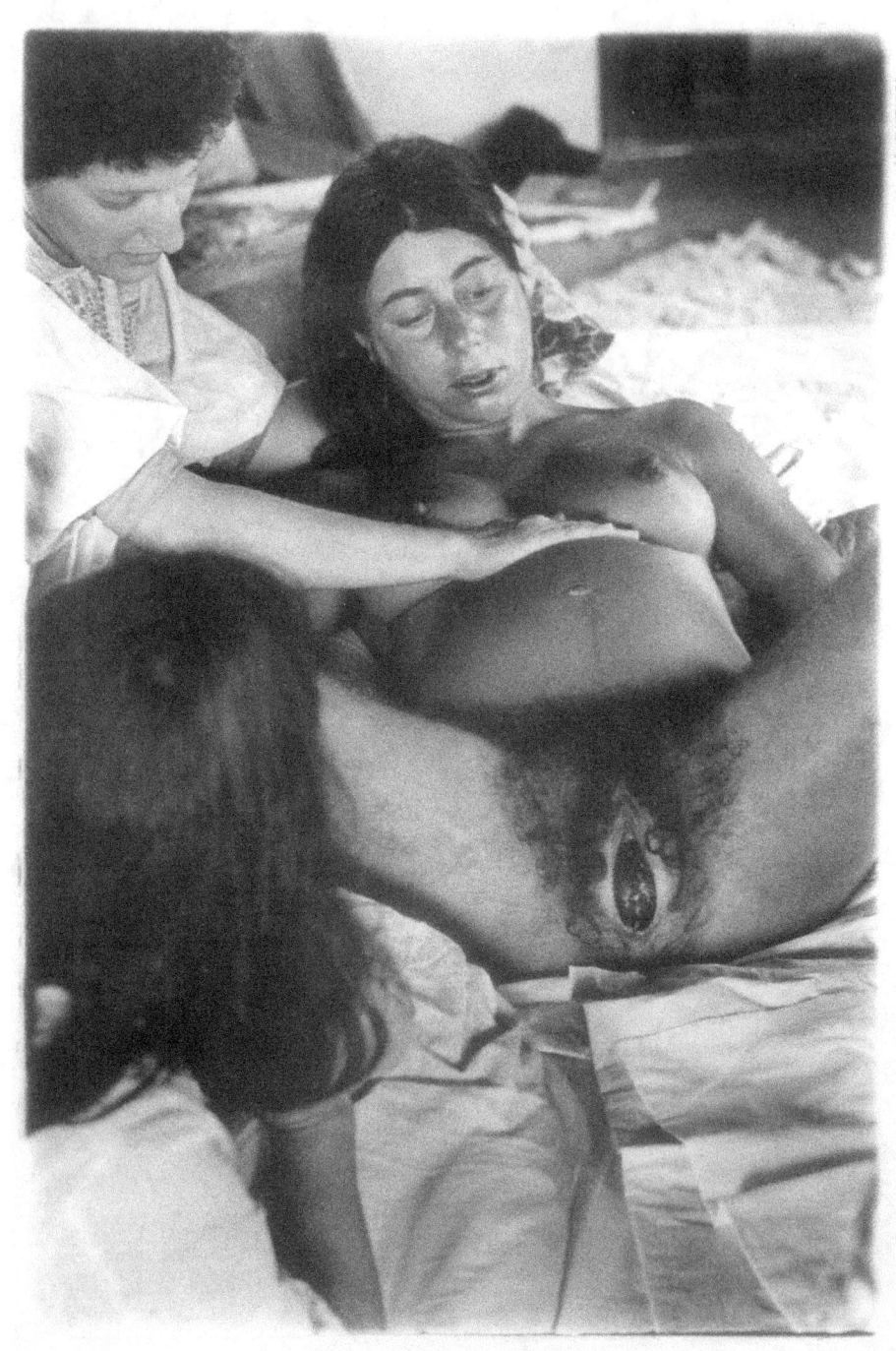

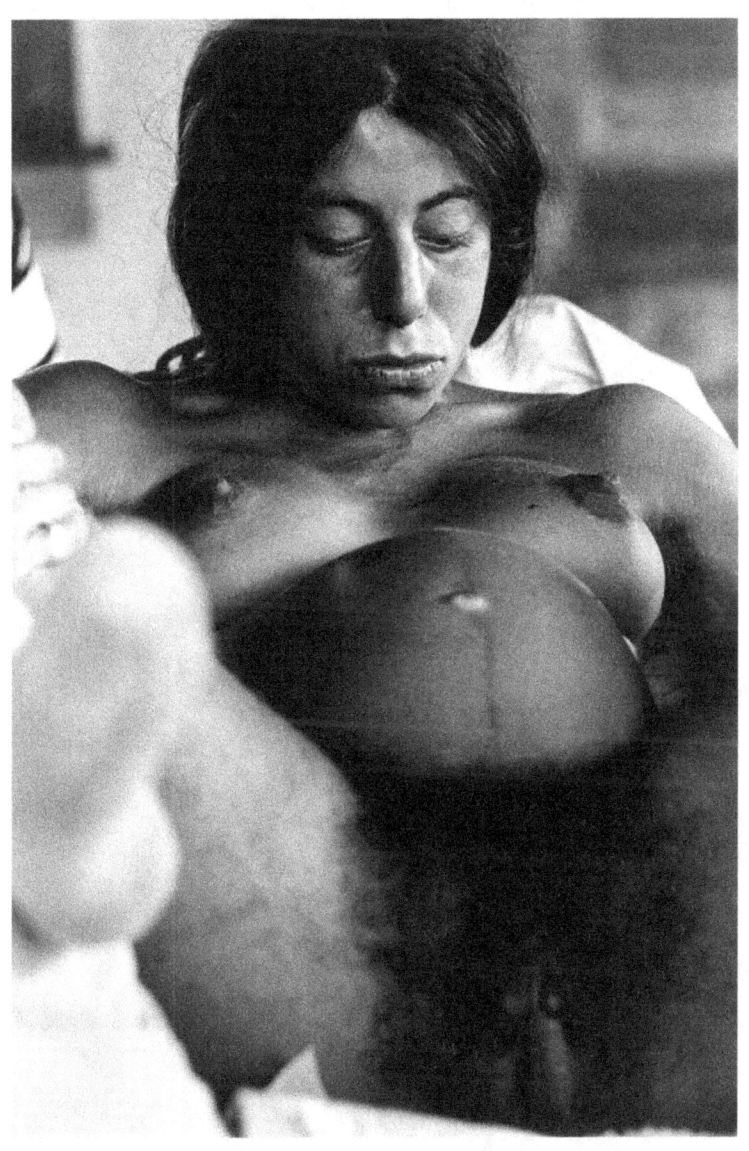

The SHMNA still being chanted:
finally the head slips past
the lips of the vagina
almost too quickly to see—
I am holding a strange dark
skinned head in my palms
his face looking upward
dark with a white sheath over it
blood spotting its crevices
the top of the head elongated
like a mushroom or the crown chakra
of a sculpted Buddha
due to its long struggle toward life—
he immediately cries and breathes
first world sound sweet and loud.
Bill cleans mucous and fluids
from nose and mouth with
sterilized aspirators;
suddenly (all of this occurring
in an eternal instant)
the next contraction ejects
his male body into my hands
with the help of a slight almost
imperceptible twist to help
its shoulders fit thru vagina.
Everyone shouts "It's a boy."
And Laurie laughs as I hand
her this tiny male being
with a Buddha crowned head
that Bill says will return
to natural shape soon—
Laurie relaxes back on the bed
baby face down on her warm belly.
We all explode in kisses and joy.

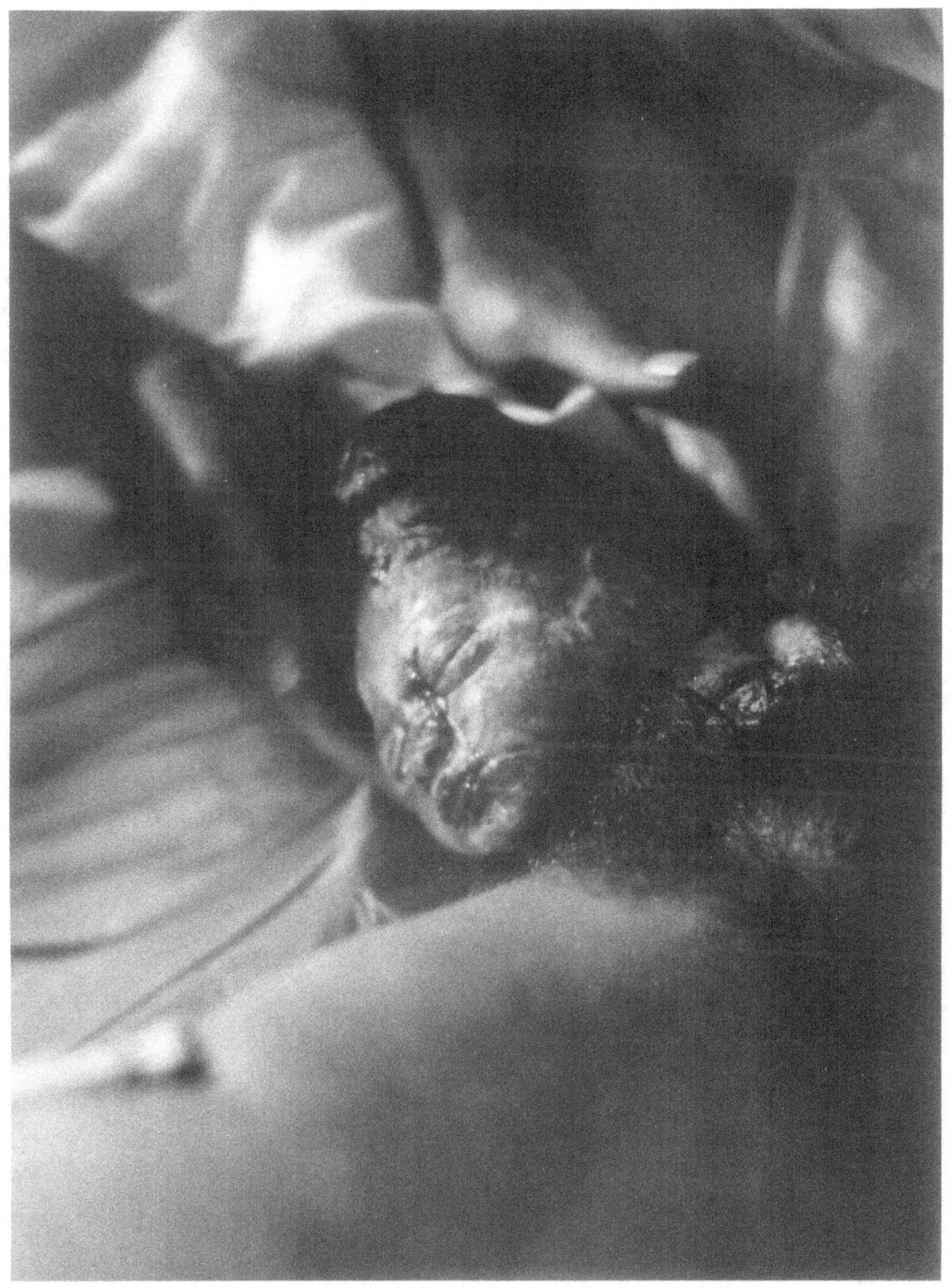

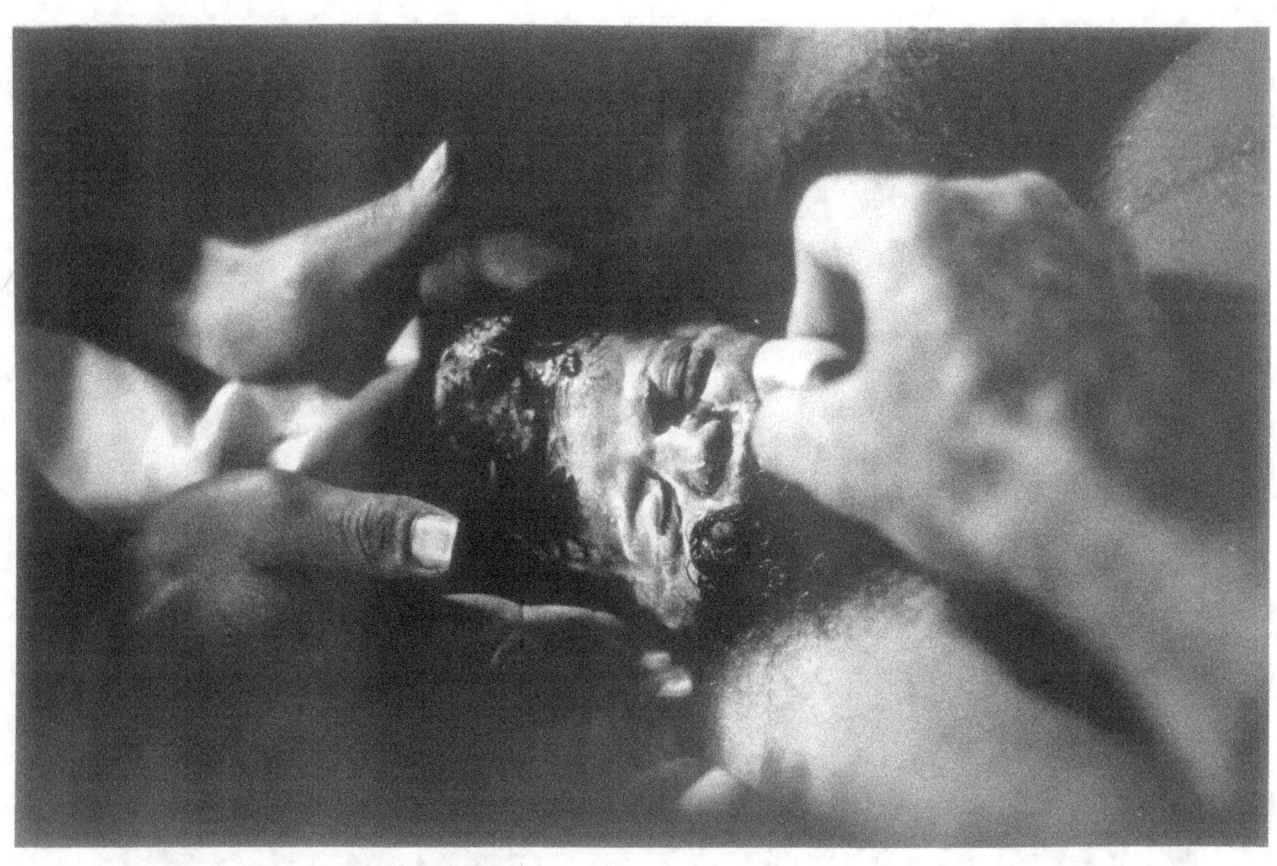

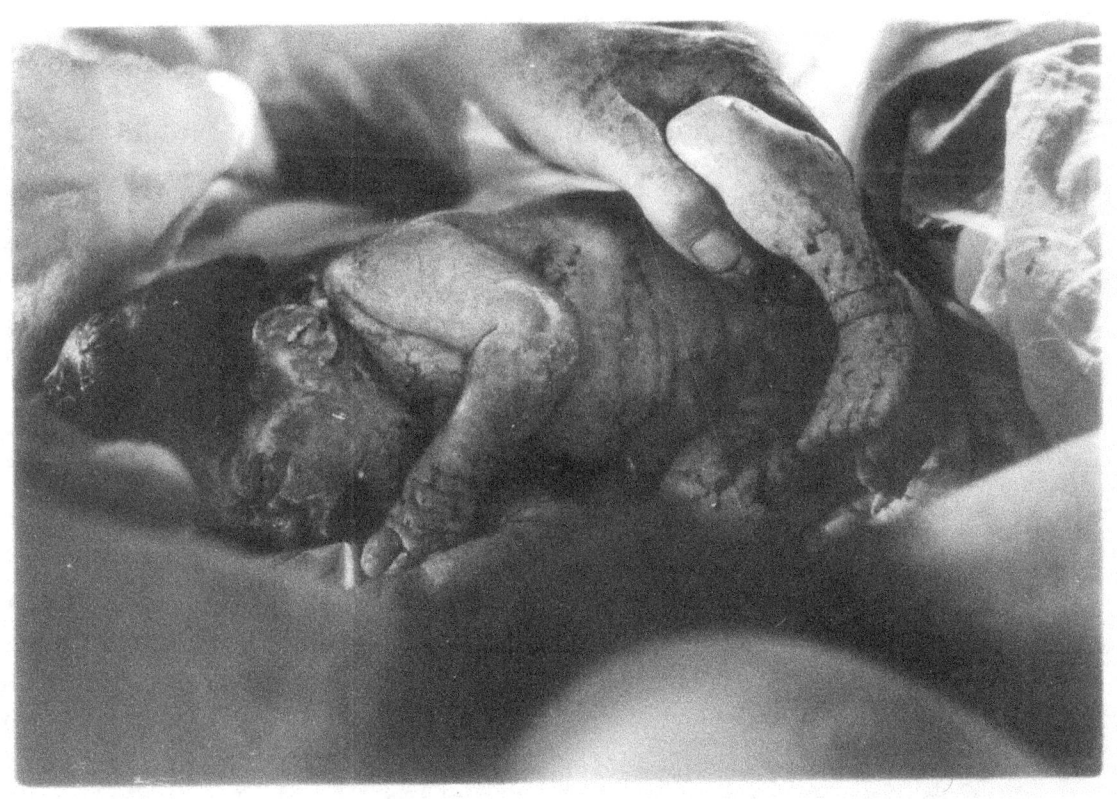

After twenty minutes or so pass
boy's head is already returning to normal shape
and we prepare to cut umbilical cord
with white shoelaces and sterilized scissor==
first we milk remnants of
rich womb food toward stomach;
then we tie tight square knot
with white shoelace in middle
of the cord between still wombed
placenta and breathing child;
second shoelace is tied
with tight square know
two inches from belly
and cut with scissor
¾ of an inch above this knot
so that the knot doesn't slip
and he is world-borne—
another unique self
launched through the mysteriously
born body onto earth-life.

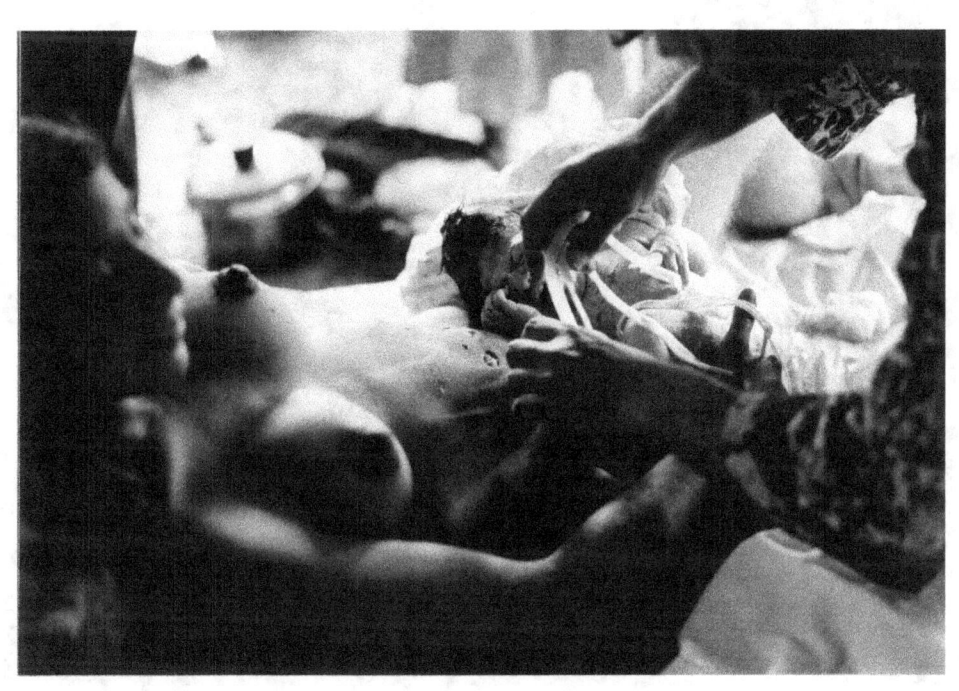

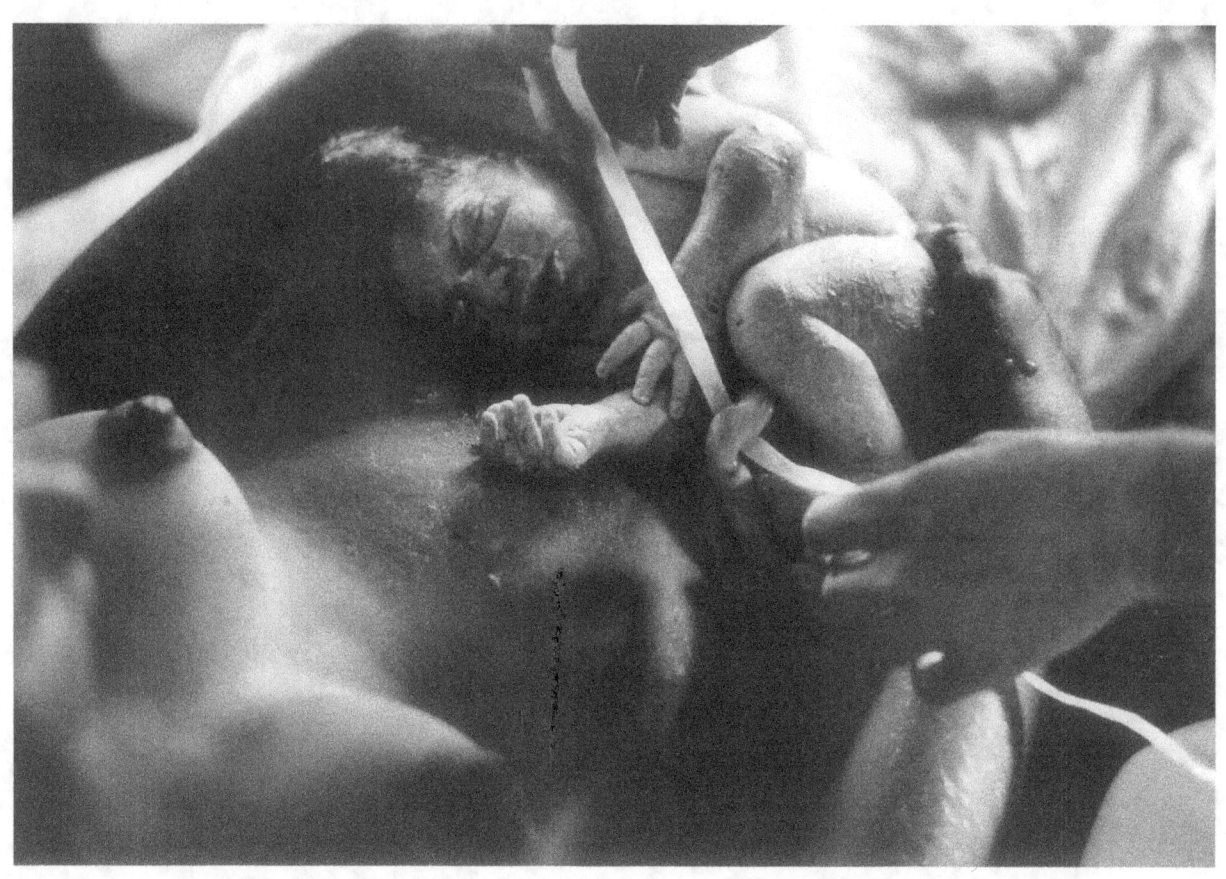

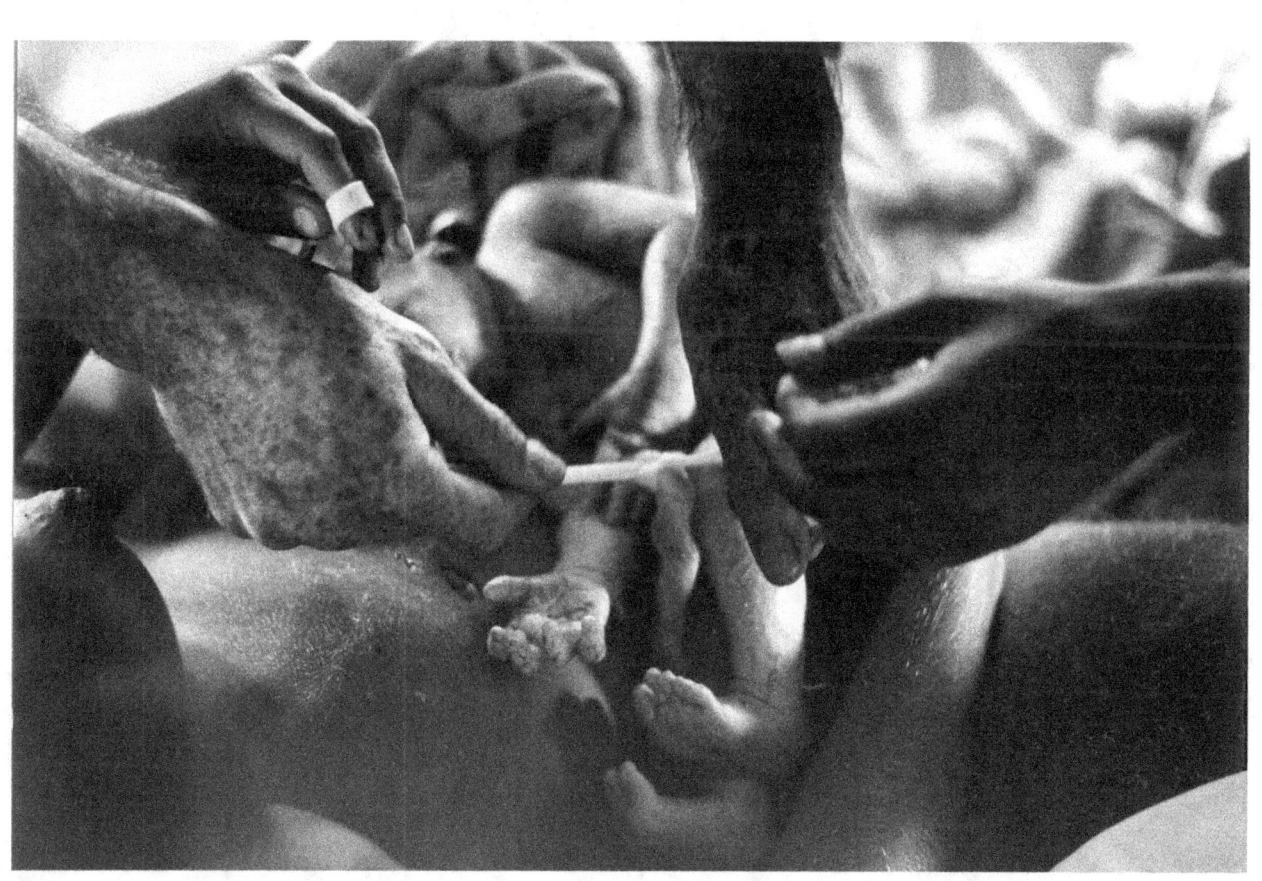

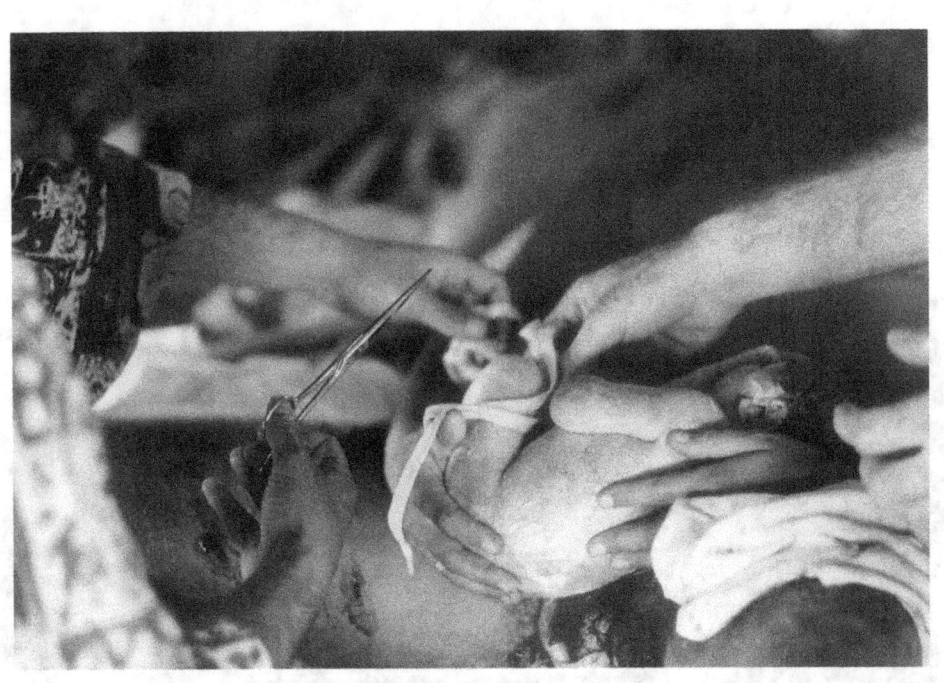

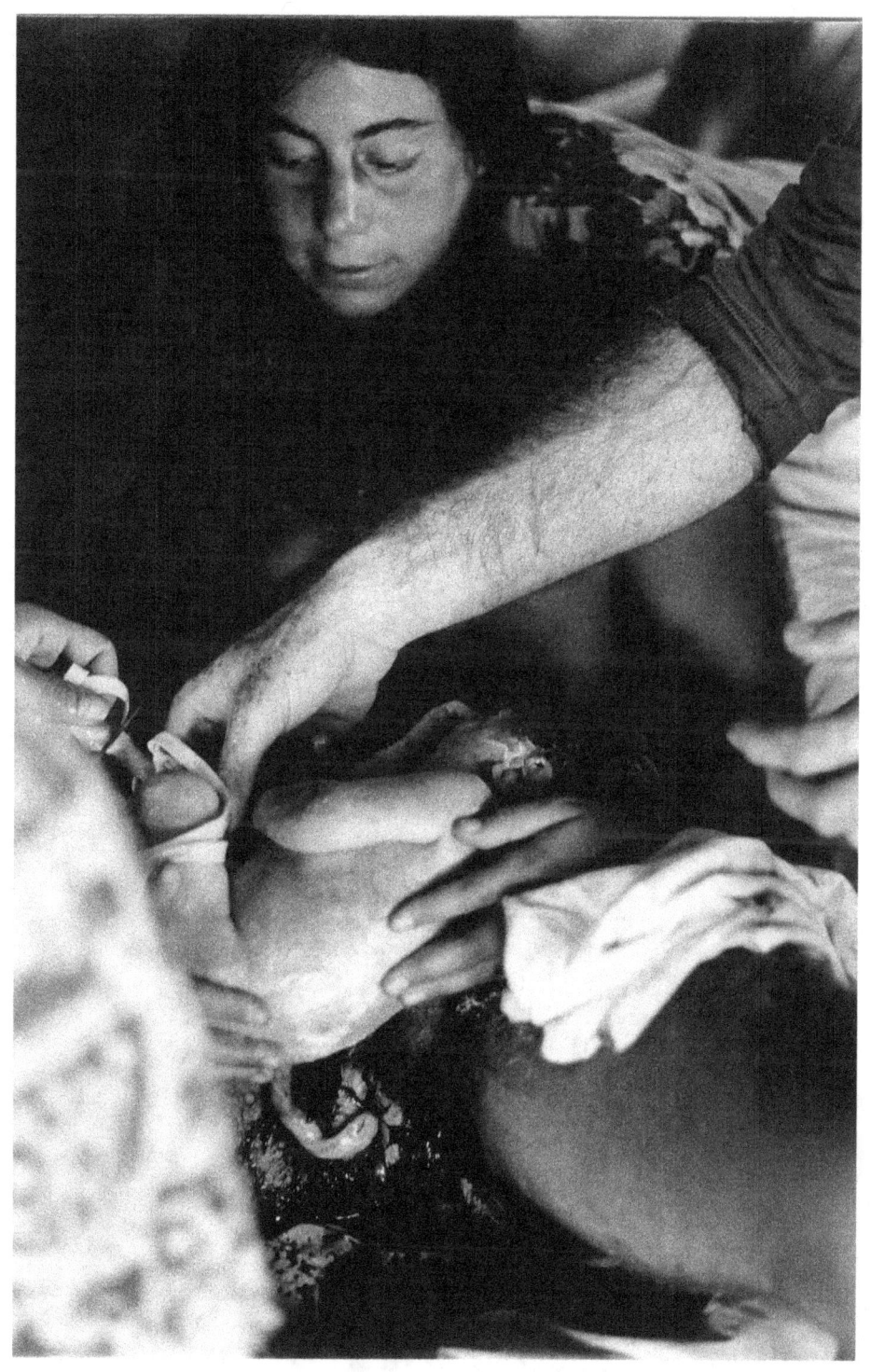

About ½ hour after birth
Laurie feels another wave
and the placenta pops from her Yanni
deep purple silken pouch
and we place it in a bowl
and offer everyone a taste
of the elixir, builder and nourisher
of bodies and I decide
to bury it in our garden
to nourish our soil—
all bed pads, sheet and
clothes are then changed
and Laurie's surface ripped perineum
is rinsed with hydrogen peroxide
and Bill says she should rinse
it every day with peroxide and open
her legs to the sun
and it will heal naturally,
(And it did.)

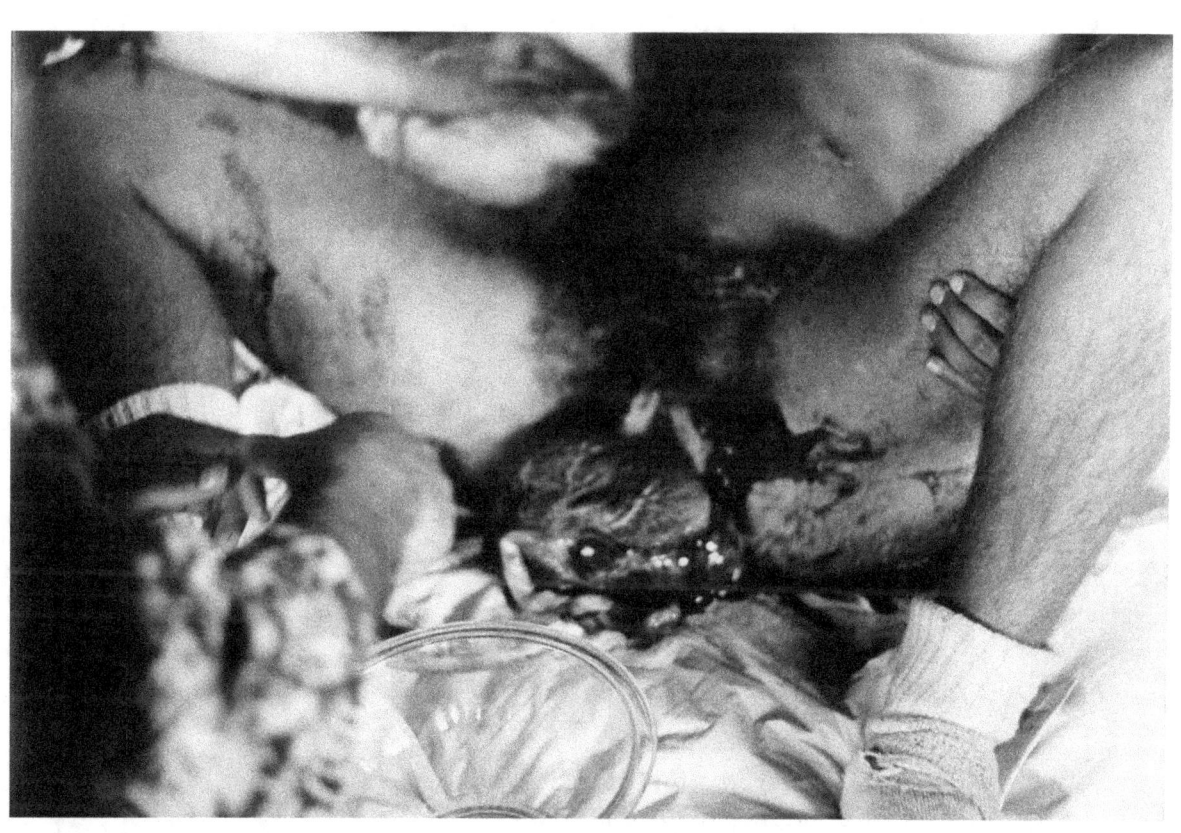

Laurie dressed now in white blouse
looking radiant names the child RIVER
and I say his second name ALBION
after the river bordering our ranch
and Blake's envisioned angel of ancient England
and Atlantis of which England was the daughter.
Someone suggest giving him a Jewish name.
and I say ELIJAH who flew
to the sun in a chariot
in love and prophecy of the ONE GOD
promising to return as messenger of Messiah.

Later Laurie and I throw coins
asking I CHING Oracle
"Who is this being that
has sprung into our midst?"
The Oracle answers TING,
The CAULDRON and from
this reading we received
our first understanding
and instructions for fostering
and nurturing this new life.
The three of us purposed
to bring light and love
to the turning planet.

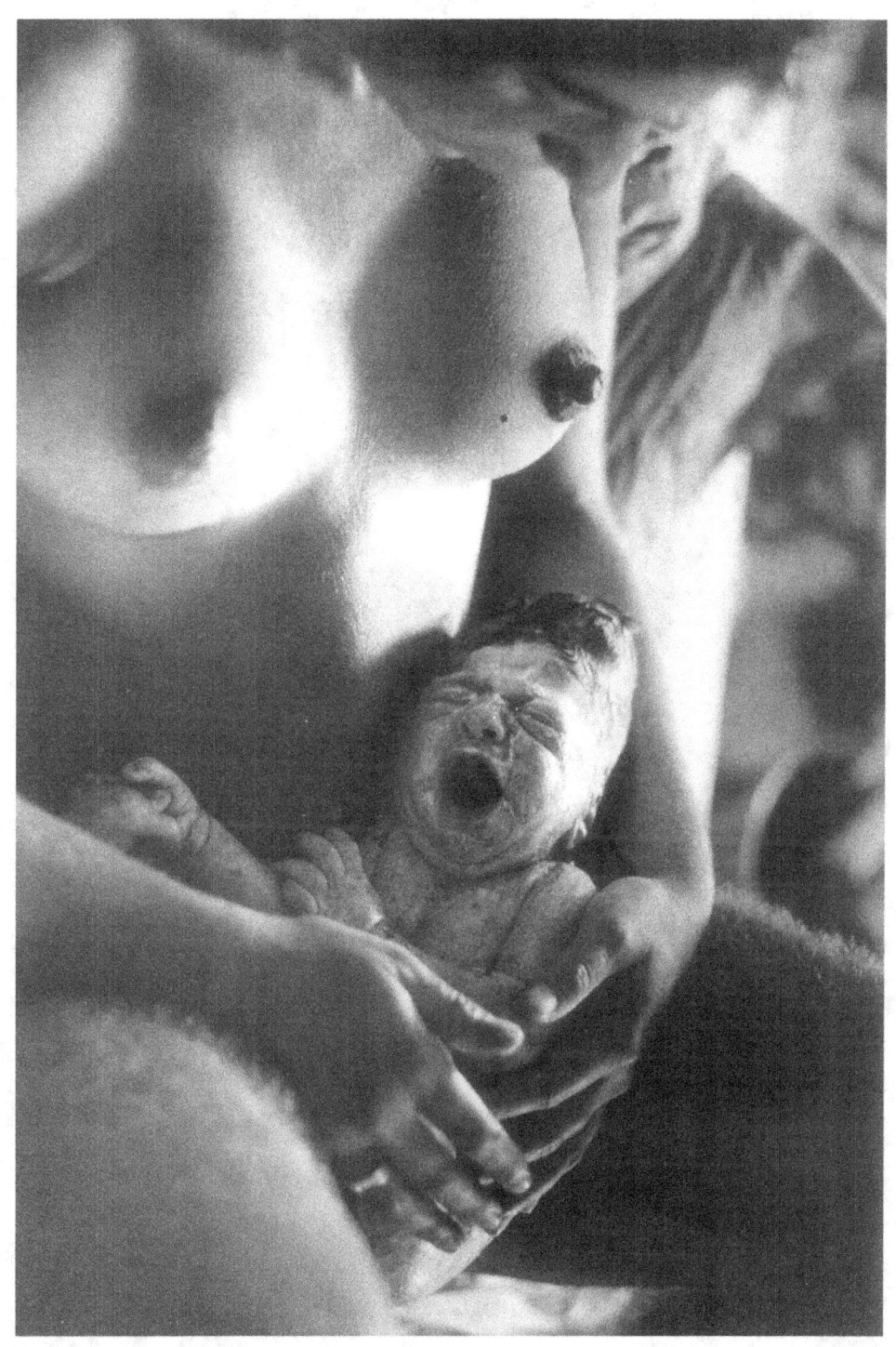

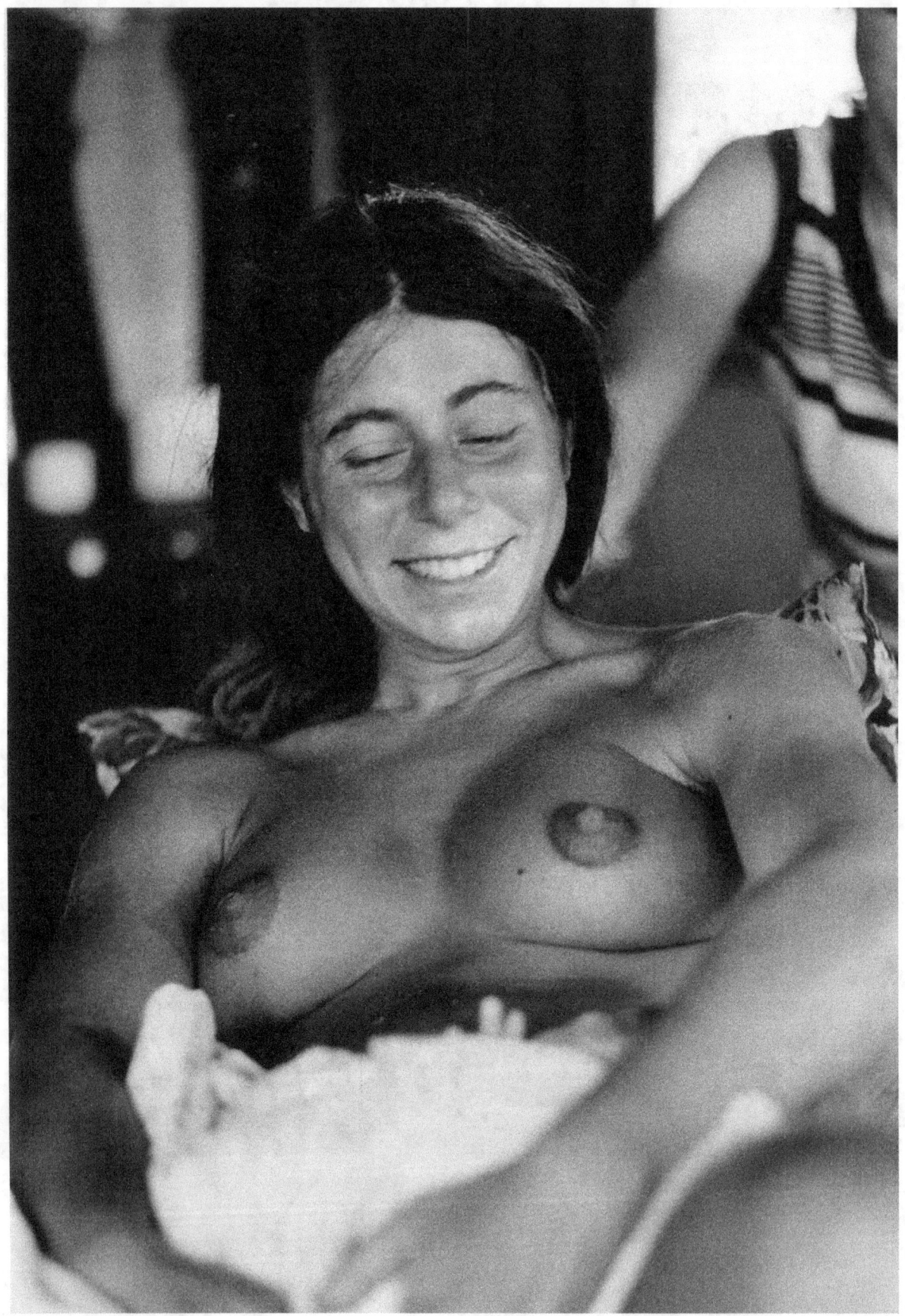

After about am hour River's
head is naturally shaped and beautiful,
his face looking like a boxer's
after a hard through victorious fight;
he is very dark and looks more
like an American Indian than a white man.
We bathe this eyes with a boric acid solution
because they are red and swollen.
We reflect that the long and hard
passage was due to his coming thru
face up instead of face down.
If we had been in a hospital
the doctors probably would have considered
the position a complication serious enough
to have used anesthetics and
delivered child with forceps.
I ask Laurie if there was any pain
and she says "No pain, but
I know what the Earth
feels like making a mountain."

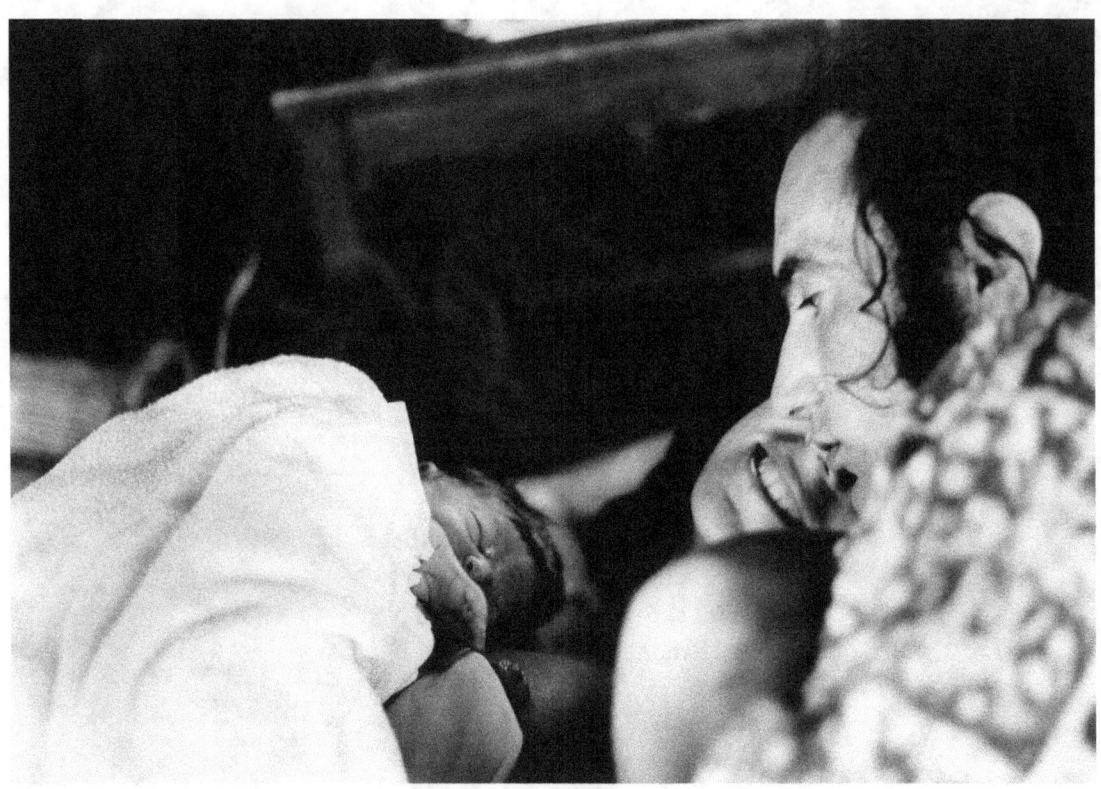

Bill Bowen and I walk
that evening down the road
under a million stars—
the Milky Way stretching
its two arms around the heavens—
we speak of the beauty
we had witnessed and the courage
of women and the leap of conscious
freedom we had shared with these women
and the harmony that passes
from the house of pleasure
into our hands when
a new person in a helpless
miniature body appears in our palm
designed with conscious intelligence
to grow and become human.

There would be no war if every man
received his son onto this planet
in this way and had known his wife
in this act of ecstasy.

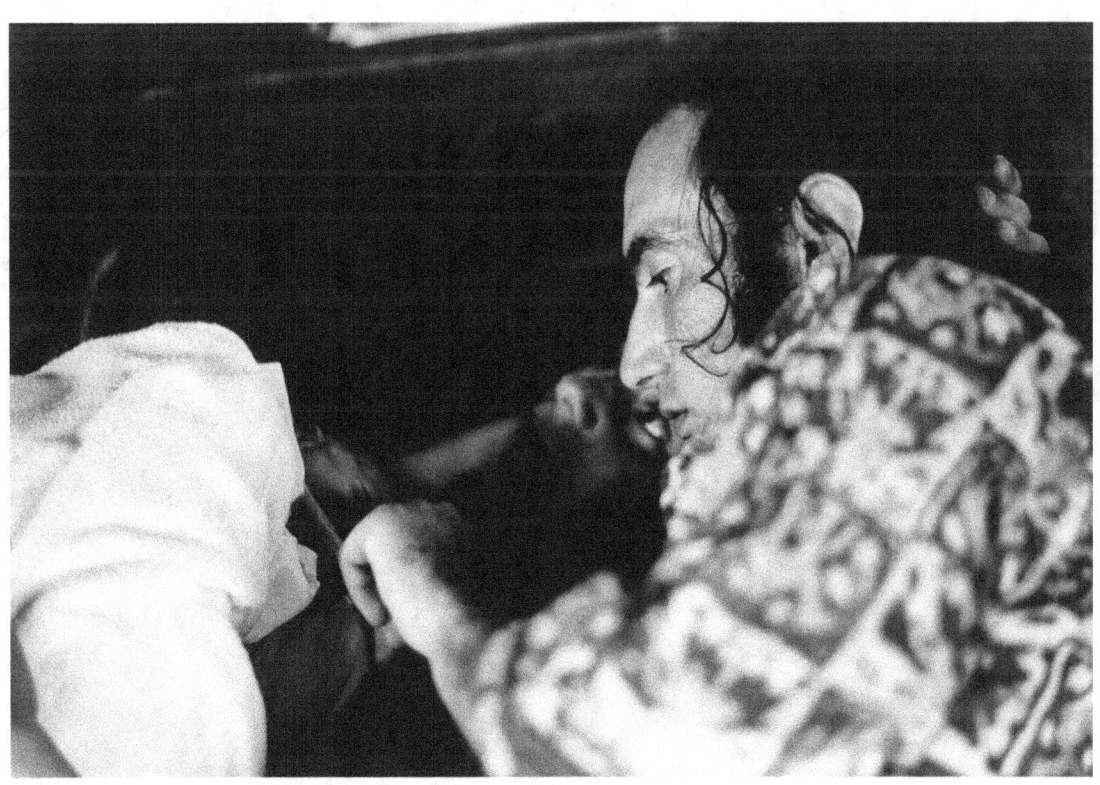

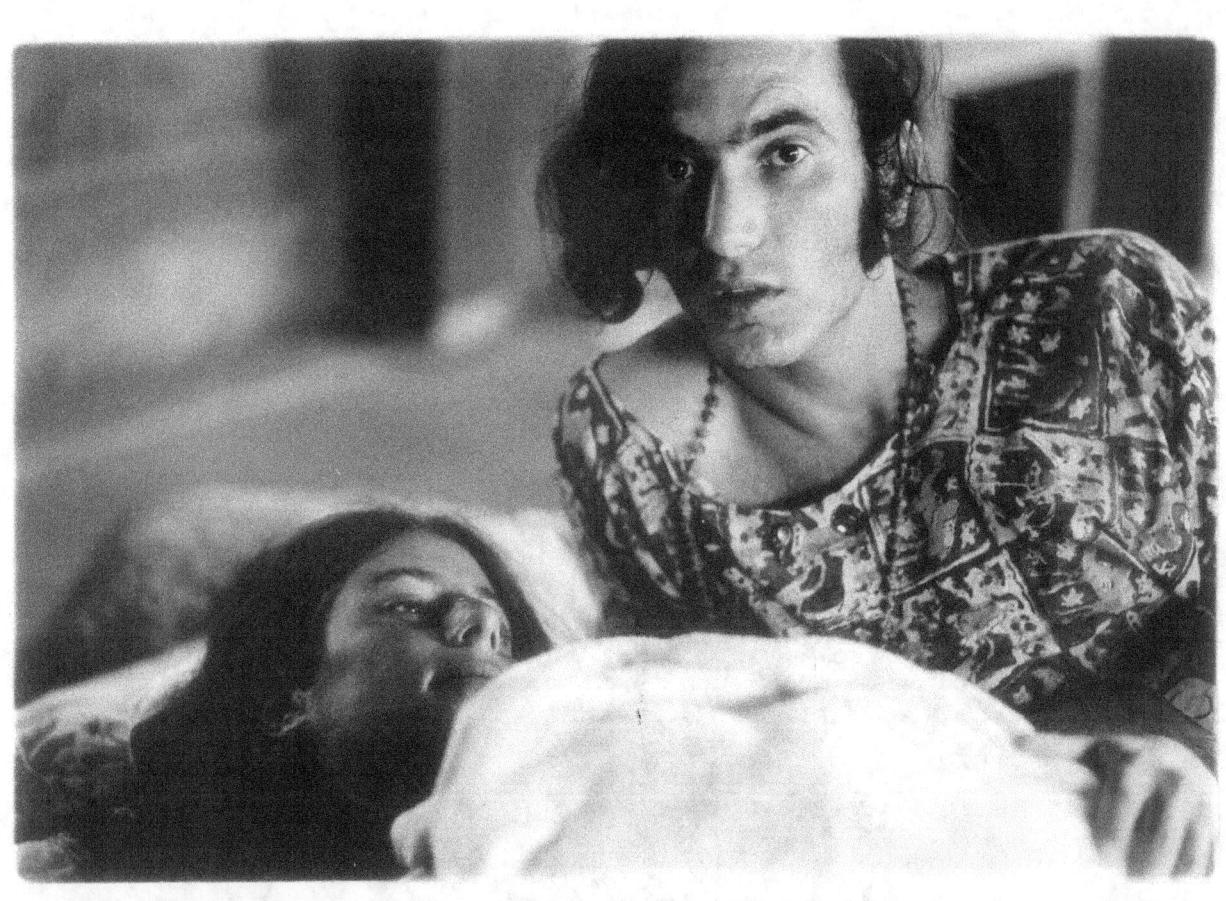

River Albion Elijah Cohen
Growing
                    likes fire
and breast of woman
has lovely round chin
perfect form
male man
He sprang from
my loins
We live in a tipi now

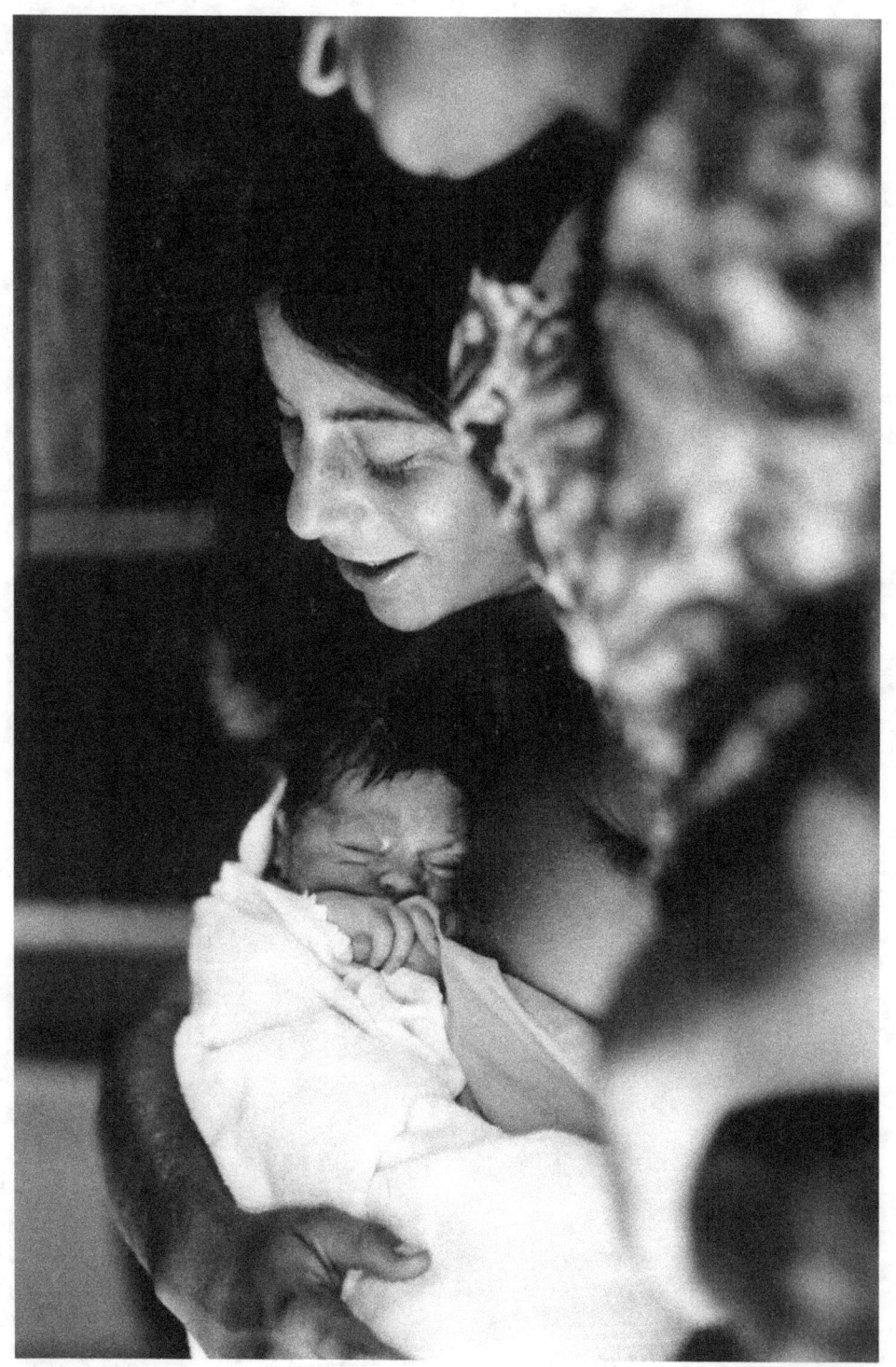

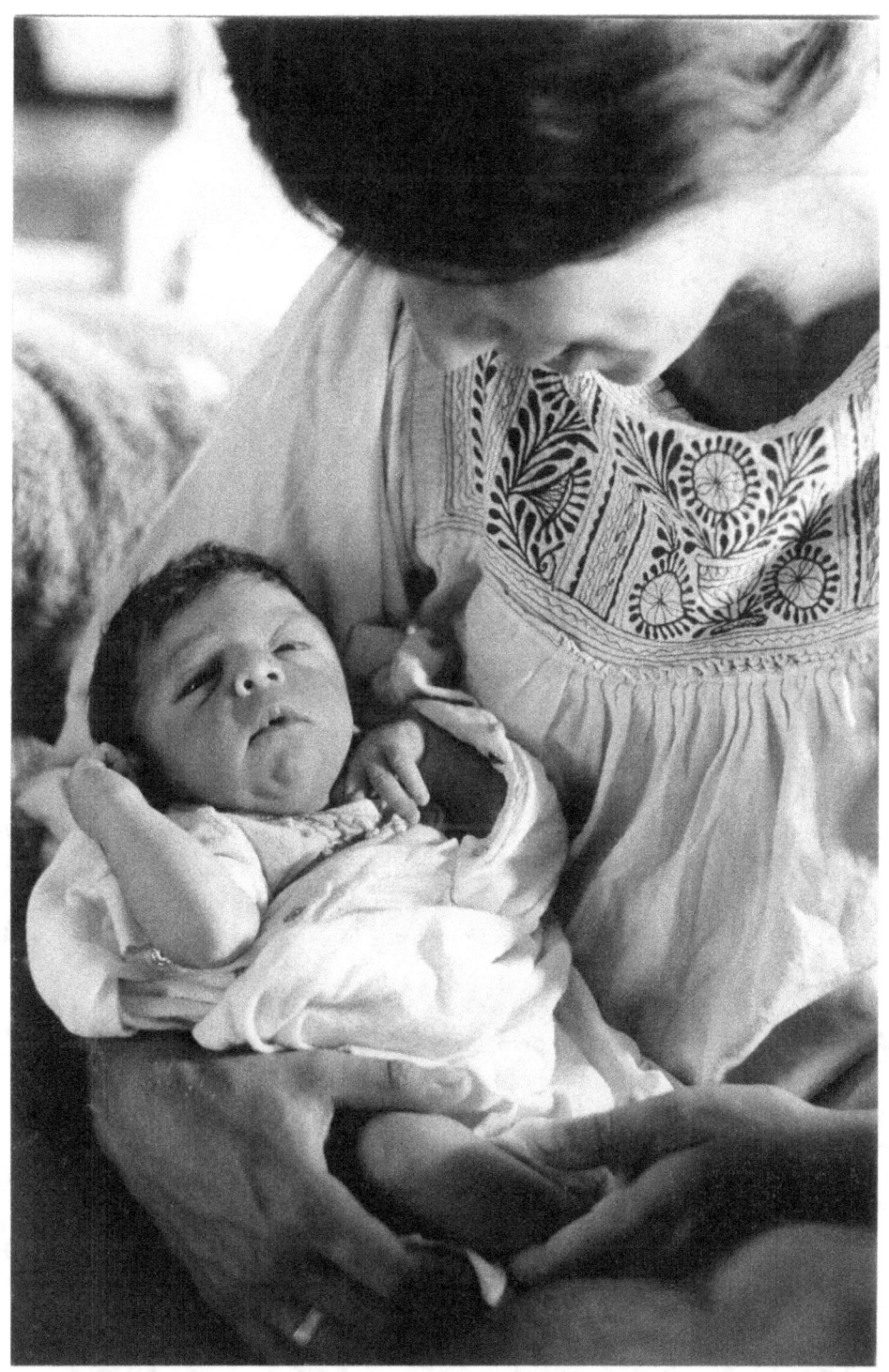

After word, purpose & worldscore

Throbbing within the pride of man in his machines and systems of political and economic control, sitting in the heart of our sorrow, causing much of the confusion, violence and inhumanity of modern life is a fundamental hatred, distrust and fear of the human body and the self or soul that inhabits that body to guide and direct each person toward his or her acts, ideals, and purposes, style of living and toward the political and economic forms he or she agrees to live within, institutionalize and support in small or large groups, that is, families, communities or nations, Many scholars like Marx, Engels, Norman Brown, Wilhelm Reich, Herbert Marcuse, Charles Fourier and a few does like A.S. Neil, founder of Summerhill, Gurdjieff, and Fritz Perls, originator of gestalt group psychotherapy and great sages like Ramakrishna, Vivekananda, Ramana
Maharshi have been exploring ways of bringing man, woman, and children into a free and joyful interaction with their own self, with each other and with their bodies.

Childbirth is the doorway into bodily life and it has been surrounded by taboo and fear for thousands of years, and western Judeo-Christian culture has especially consigned women and the birth process to disapproval and distrust, thereby scarring our conscious-ness against life from its very inception. No wonder we are shadows on the screen of sorrow and yearn for the touch of love – we have yet to come alive and trust our bodies and allow our minds and hearts their natural and expanding freedom.

The purpose of making this personal experience of childbirth public is to eradicate the fear of childbirth from the minds of men and women – the presence of this fear brings anxiety and tension to the mine and body and this anticipation is the cause of the pain women experience during the childbirth process. This predisposition to fear-tension-pain is also the cause of many of the complications sometimes experienced in the process such long labors and hemorrhages.

Birth is a Norman process, as normal process, as normal and precoded into humans as digestion through more intense and dramatic. Ninety-six percent of all childbirth is without complications to either mother or child. Of the other four percent, many are minor complications that can be dealt with by being patient and letting the process go on without too much interference or anxiety plus some knowledge of what can be expected and what can be done under unusual or unexpected circumstances. This knowledge can be acquired by research of direction from experienced and relatively unstructured doctors who are interested in a humanization of the birth process and from experienced midwives.

Many birth complications would be eliminated by replacing confidence and knowledge about childbirth where fear, taboo and ignorance held sway. A bibliography of books on natural childbirth written by medical men who have gathered experiences and methods for attaining painless and relaxed birth experiences is included at the end of this book.

This book though it tries to convey as much as the poet could recreate and the photographer could photograph is not a manual of directions by a woman who is pregnant or a man or woman who wants to attend, witness or aid as midwife in order to reorient oneself to original instinctual naturalness of the birth experience. It is easy and life enhancing to attain this reorientation. Briefly, a woman should be of good general health, have her own and father's blood type determined to Rh Factor, and establish a healthy balanced diet, give up smoking cigarettes, and should choose to read one of the books about Natural Childbirth in order to develop a knowledge of what is happening to her body during pregnancy and childbirth and to learn breathing techniques and exercises. Tribal communication with women who have delivered naturally gives confidence and guidance. For those who would attend a homebirth knowledge of pregnancy, the female body and childbirth should be gained by reading a book about Natural Childbirth and those on midwifery, as well as speaking with a sympathetic doctor and those who have attended births at home. Remember the ocean of bliss, wisdom and existence which we are and have always been and will always be prepare for childbirth in that light with your loved ones. For those who are inwardly and mentally free from fear, this book will be helpful; for those who are unsure, it might be inspirational.

Through most births are normal and natural there are some that can be aided by experienced doctors and/ or midwives, some by modern medical and surgical techniques in hospitals. For example, women whose pelves are very small as determined by pelvic examination should be delivered in a hospital; unless there is a very experienced midwife, multiple births should be delivered by a doctor and if he so desires, in a hospital; a child who is in breech position in the womb should be delivered by a very experienced midwife or doctor either at home or hospital at their discretion. These examples are rare and constitute less than four percent of all childbirths and mostly can be diagnosed during the pregnancy period.

There is some very small risk in childbirth of unexpected injury or death, but the risk is there as a natural factor whether in a hospital or at home, whether with doctors or midwife or tribe or just husband or even alone. There are the rare occurrences like hemorrhaging that could be aided more quickly if a woman was in a hospital or was serviced by a mobile childbirth units as in England. But there are also occurrences in hospitals like exposure to diseases and the general fear-tension-pain-sickness atmosphere of hospital birth that would be prevented if childbirth was approached as a natural, ecstatic and supportive experience. Of the 20 nations that record mortality rates in childbirth, America, where most births are in hospitals, has the second most deaths in childbirth. So I feel that the psychological and spiritual preparation for childbirth on the part of mothers and those who are there to support her with knowledge, love, trust and beauty are the most important factors in successful, painless and ecstatic childbirth.

II

Why suddenly in the midst of massive trepidation over population explosion are we confronted with a book praising and glorifying childbirth?

First and out front, this was Laurie's and five other women's experience, while I was present as witness, comforted and mid-husband. The birth experience, though primarily a woman's adventure, reorients and turns the mind toward new possibilities and awareness of life. So this is a presentation of our adventure in authentic living; an ancient experience that is new for our time and place.

Secondly, these births were experienced within cooperative earth based communities – non-hierarchical, unsalaried, voluntary groups held together by mutual help and sharing of resources and land. This supportive volunary environment under the non-exploited wing of mother nature in a primary heart to heart interweaving of people allows the greatest opportunity for the growth of both freedom and interactive responsibility. In groups similar to this (though more sophisticated and evolved) this continent was inhabited for at least 5000 years by the American Indian without overpopulation or exploitation of resources like water, wood, wildlife and metals, without much war, or sickness either of soul, mind, or body.

We feel that overpopulation and food scarcity is based from India to America on an inequitable distribution and private ownership of land which leads to sustaining personal greed and ambition of the few and the oppression of many, which circumstance forces the people into completely chaotic, unplanned and useless cities to live lives of poverty, boredom, sickness, psychological and spiritual despair. out of contact with earth based tribal heritage which is everyone's by virtue of being planet born.

American land has been and will be shared and worked communally again soon in either small or large village or tribal groups without rents or crop payoffs and the resultant insecurity of landlordism which is the burden of most of the people of the world – hitched to the rich man's wagon. The necessity is thereby created to reproduce many times in order to pay the landlord's dues either by work, beggary or the prostitution of daughters in order to try to lift the patriarchal, alienated, atomized, radically unsocial and unorganized family, inhabiting either tiny hut or apartments or tenant farm, out of degenerating poverty, oppression and aloneness.

The pay to live-work to pay syndrome whose backbone is the convention of the alienated, separate, disassociated patriarchal family (Backed by state and church patriarchate authority) can be passed through and transcended by holding all thing in common in communal or village or tribal groups either religiously or culturally or work oriented, living on the fertile productive Mother Planet, sharing intimately in all fife's joys and sorrows, experimenting with other forms of sexual relationship and family and child rearing and pooling all the energies and talent of individuals into effective pleasurable work and learning, and by expansion of life consciousness through interpersonal barrier burstings and mergings of human rhythm with planet rhythm. Thus providing new potentials in spiritual, ecological and technological modes – experiments for the new age are well under way in Outer Mongolia, China, Israel, the American commune movement, and the Isle of Pines in Cuba.

This is not to put down chemical or mechanical or surgical or medical means of birth control for those who want them not for those who want to forcefully impose them (for those who want to save the world and feed the people by forcefully imposing birth control, they might try their hand at controlling the birth patterns and man's uses of thirteen billion domestic animal that man supports and feeds on grains and pasture). The problem is immense and immediate but social reorganization and land reform along the lines of small group direct democracy, group erotic freedom, and pleasurable useful and life enhancing work (like planning and building your own environment, and experimenting with new social forms) must go hand in hand with birth control in order to bring in underdeveloped countries (their unholy alliance is the cross and bones know as imperialism). The fear that there is too little for too many increases the blind urge to increase their military power and material possessions and resources. This fear is the background of the falsified differences between ideologies which confront a capitalism that is state corporatism and communism that is also state corporatism. The broader aspects of the oneness that is the planetary circumstance that we are all in the same kettle of blue-green soup fails to effect or increase the compassion, love and selflessness of world leaders in particular, but also the people of the world in order to energetically work toward environmental and social change, and to research new and cleaner energy sources such as magnetic and solar energies and to study changes in land use and animal use (especially in terms of meat eating) and agricultural and cultural attitudes. Most of the people of the developed countries are either ignorant of the immediacy of the problem or are hypnotized by their leaders and media into senseless consumption of world resources, interpersonal fear and conflict and criminal waste. So we are trying to affect consciousness toward releasing more compassion, love, simplicity and fearlessness into the world we and our children will love to preserve and improve.

Items for Ceremonial Childbirth at Home

1. Clean room with disinfectant soap.

2. Prepare ceremonial clothes for attendant, mother and baby – sterilize and store.

3. Sheet – sterilized.

4. Scissor – sterilized by boiling.

5. Two white shoelaces – sterilized by boiling.

6. Nose and mouth rubber aspirators – sterilized by boiling.

7. Phisohex soap and boiled water for washing.

8. Sponge – small piece for mother to suck on when mouth is dry.

9. Disposable bed pads or newspapers for keeping delivery area clean.

10. Towel or diapers for washing – sterilized.

11. Boric acid or silver nitrate – for protection against passing on venereal disease to newborn.

12. Kotex – super.

13. Incense.

14. Music – hand drum, flute, guitar.

15. Altar – fire earth air water.

Bibliography

The best method is probably to pick one of these books and let its knowledge become part of your own – then your instincts will take over from there.

PAINLESS CHILDBIRTH – THANK YOU DR. LAMAZE
by Majorie Karmel; Dolphin Books, Doubleday & Company, Inc., Garden City, New York, (paperback)

THE NEW CHILDBIRTH
by Erna Wright; Hart Publishing Company, Inc., New York City, (paperback)

CHILDBIRTH: A MANUAL FOR PRIGNANCY AND DELIVERY
by John S. Miller, M.D.; Atheneum Publishers, 1963.

CHILDBIRTH WITHOUT FEAR
by Grantly Dick Read; Harper & Brothers, 1954.

AWAKE & AWARE
by Erwin Chabon; Delacorte Press

Midwifery

PREGNANCY, CHILDBIRTH AND THE NEWBORN: A manual for Rural Midwives
by Eloesser, Galt and Hemingway; Instituto Indigenista Interamericano,
Nino Heroes, 139, Mexico 7, D.F., 1959. (second English Edition)

EMERGENCY CHILDBIRTH –A Manual
by Gregory J. White, M.D.; Police Training Foundation, 3412 Ruby St.,
Franklin Park, Illinois 60131.